MICHAEL STENNING

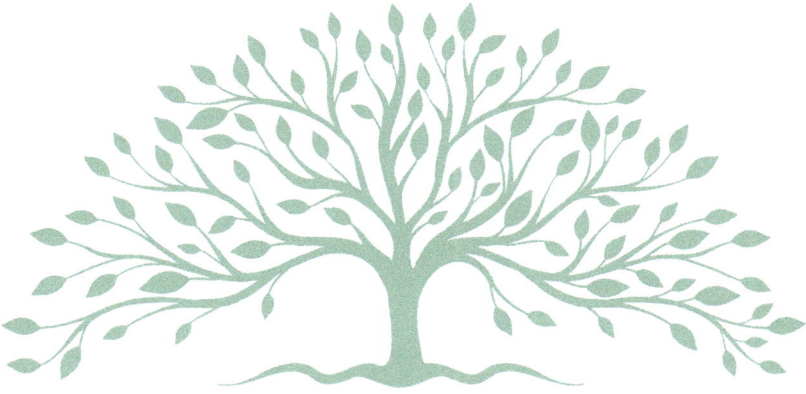

Embodying Practice

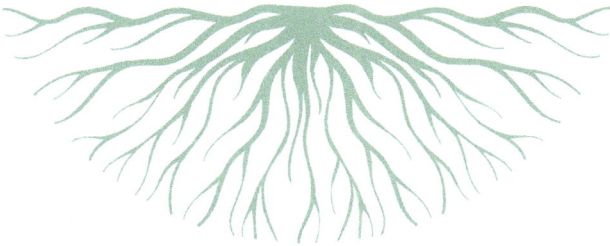

A guide for new teachers
of the Alexander Technique

First published in 2025 by Freedom in Action Pty Ltd.

A catalogue record for this book is available from the National Library of Australia at catalogue.nla.gov.au.

Cover and internal design and layout by Tess McCabe.

Illustrations by Robert Clode.

All web addresses are current at time of writing.

Paperback ISBN: 978-1-7641785-0-1

Ebook ISBN: 978-1-7641785-1-8

www.freedominaction.com.au

DISCLAIMER
The views, opinions and thoughts expressed in this book belong solely to the author and are intended for the purpose of education and reflection. This book should not be used as a substitute for professional assistance, therapeutic support or medical advice. In the event of physical or mental distress, please consult with appropriate health professionals. The application of ideas and information presented in this book is the choice of the reader, who assumes full responsibility for their understanding, interpretation or results. The author assumes no responsibility for the actions or choices of any reader.

A teacher must continue to be a learner, always enlivening their personal practice of the Alexander Technique. How do we keep reinspiring ourselves and renewing our curiosity and excitement?

Contents

Preface

As a new Alexander teacher in 1985, I had many things to learn and would have appreciated guidance. Over thirty years later, in a plenary session at the 2018 International Alexander Technique Congress, the audience was asked who among them had felt confident and competent to teach when they had finished their teacher training. I was surprised to learn that well over half of those present had not felt ready to teach when their trainers had finished with them.

Over many years of running professional development courses for Alexander Technique teachers, I have noticed that some teachers continue to lack confidence, and there are areas of the Technique that they may not be clear about. One area concerns an appreciation of how (or even that) their legs fit into the picture of going up, the primary control and working with their directions. Of course, lip service may be paid, for example, by saying, 'Knees forward and away.' But in actuality, the legs may effectively be missing, together with the deeply consequential effect of enlivening the legs: fuller integration of all the primary control relationships.

The second area is what first-generation teacher Margaret Goldie referred to as 'brain work'. Many find it difficult to trust the directions and the process of directing. Often, a little hedging of bets goes on: at the same time as giving directions, we want to know that our directions are having an effect, i.e., we want to feel them out or even do them. This is, of course, self-limiting.

The third area that recurs is the importance of continuously and joyfully recommitting to the basics of inhibition and direction as a means of moving through difficulties. All our activities and other disciplines may inform our practice of the Alexander Technique, but there has to be a practice. How this practice manifests is, of course, purely personal and subjective. The rigour and discipline instilled during one's teacher training should play a role in shaping it.

Having been struck by these observations, I have been moved to try to address them, and this volume is the result. This book is intended to support trainees and new teachers, and to encourage an ongoing process of building understanding, skill and confidence among teachers at all levels of experience. I hope that you find it helpful.

Just before I qualified, my head of training, Jeanne Haahr (Day), said to my class, 'You know more than your pupil.' This is true. Trust in the Technique, in time, in the discipline of learning, in yourself, and in the absolute basics of inhibition and direction. Apply these fundamentals and watch the process unfold.

Overview

The thing to be known grows with the knowing.

NAN SHEPHERD[1]

What follows is a set of reflections on the process of skill-building in learning and teaching the Alexander Technique. I share observations, clarify definitions, illuminate technicalities and elucidate process. I offer an overview while also highlighting necessary detail. I cover what I consider basic learning for any trainee teacher, which can be refined and deepened over a lifetime of engagement. Certain sections may have more relevance for some readers than others. Chapter 4: 'General specifics and practical explorations' includes some explorations of traditional ways of working. Whatever I offer rests on what I have learnt from my teachers and decades of my own practice.

---

1   Nan Shepherd, *The Living Mountain* (Canongate Books [Kindle], 2011).

This book is not intended for newcomers to the Alexander Technique. The extent of experience of readers may vary widely. You could be a trainee teacher, a newly qualified teacher, a teacher who sees just a few pupils a week, a teacher returning to teaching after a break, or an experienced teacher perhaps wanting to revisit some basics or looking for stimulation. Whichever you are, I trust that this book will provide some food for thought. My background is in music, and so I include some musical analogies. You will find there is repetition of ideas and Alexander directions, which occurs as a consequence of context within the book. These chapters may be dipped into rather than necessarily read sequentially.[2]

For someone who practises the Alexander Technique, learning is open-ended: you start with your first private lesson or group class and keep learning as you continue having lessons and beyond. This means that you apply the Alexander Technique in your life, which is another way of saying that you work on yourself. As you do so, you add lived depth to your understanding. Carolyn Nicholls eloquently expressed that learning the Alexander Technique is a process of revisiting the same things repeatedly, but at a higher level, and with greater insight, each time.[3] Carolyn used the metaphor of a spiral staircase. You think you have 'got it'—understood or mastered something—until you reach such a point again, maybe a year or two or ten later, but at a higher turn of the spiral. Now you have got it. This happens again and again—each time you have got it more deeply or clearly. It is a process of deepening

---

2   Cross-references to various sections within this book are included in footnotes, using single quotes, along with a page number.

3   Carolyn Nicholls, "Analysis of the Specialised Use of the Hands in Alexander Technique Teaching" (MA diss., University of East London, 2003), 8.

your understanding of basic principles or words you thought you had already understood. For teachers, this exemplifies the continuity between learning and teaching. Without continuing to evolve your own practice of the Alexander Technique, continuing to 'move up the spiral',[4] you run the risk of stagnating. A teacher must continue to be a learner.

On being awarded a teaching certificate, a trainee is deemed to have an adequate level of basic competence in teaching. The lifelong work on the self continues. The working life of an Alexander Technique teacher is lonely in a sense, because your stock-in-trade is effectively the solo enterprise of your ability to continue to work on yourself. This applies to anyone 'living' the Alexander Technique. Living it is an internal process that manifests only in the moment. It is not like the visual arts, where you can hang your finished work on the wall and then stop thinking about it. Over time, it can be hard to maintain enthusiasm and interest in practising the Technique: you can get stuck or stale and you can encounter different or more refined versions of the same old problems. You might at times appear to have gone as far as you can with the Alexander Technique and you may lose that original spark of excitement and curiosity. At such moments, you might become interested in some other system or method, as the Alexander Technique appears no longer to 'open out'. But as a teacher, you need to be able to move past these inevitable 'choke points': where you feel you are not making progress, where you struggle to apply the Technique in your life, or where you seem to have arrived at a 'cul-de-sac' in your use, and perceive no path for further growth. These hurdles can arise at any time in your life, whether or not you are teaching the Alexander Technique. Yet if you don't continue to work on yourself, you may never find

---

4   This is a paraphrase of Carolyn Nicholls' metaphor.

out what you are capable of. It's about staying with the process, not reaching the end. How do you keep working on yourself, reinspiring yourself and renewing your personal practice?

What is it that we like about the Alexander Technique?

What do we get out of the Alexander Technique? What are the Alexander Technique goodies? It is helpful to remind ourselves of this from time to time. Answers vary and here's mine: agency. The Alexander Technique empowers me—it puts me in my own 'driver's seat'. I can make conscious choices in how I respond to life's challenges, rather than being run by routine and unconscious habit. This provides a raft of other benefits:

· As we learn to control our reactions to life's stimuli, we feel calmer and more centred;
· We may experience a sense of wholeness or integration;
· In addition, the Alexander Technique improves our physical well-being: as we breathe better and move better, we feel good. We may also look better as a consequence;
· Pain may become controllable, diminish or go away entirely;
· We learn to pay attention to and consider more deeply the array of sensory inputs we experience.

In short, we learn to use our selves better.

Why read on?

Considering familiar concepts in a different way can shine a new light on them. No matter your level of experience, I ask you to pause and question your assumptions about Alexander Technique concepts in the light of how they are presented here. The point is to question your assumptions. Indeed, they might all be in order, and re-examining may yield no further nuances. Yet it is a worthwhile exercise in affirming your path. On the other hand, as you check your assumptions now and again, it can be surprising how much a reassessment can re-enliven your practice. Anyone working with Alexander Technique principles will be learning not only for the reasons given earlier, but also for the sake of learning itself. Developing your understanding and skills is interesting, enriching and enlivening. If you are also giving lessons to paying pupils, it is more fulfilling both for you and your pupils if you continue to develop and refine your understanding and teaching skills to be an ever-better teacher. This means regularly re-examining the familiar and renewing your curiosity and excitement.

Committing for the long term: Keeping it alive

No matter how or when you begin learning the Alexander Technique, the longer you explore it, the deeper your questions can be about the what, why and how of it. Wherever you are along the path of improving the use of your self, and communicating that path to others, you are continuing to learn. You learn a set of skills, you refine them and you continue to deepen your knowledge and understanding in the process.

The basis of all these skills is that of paying attention to yourself in a way that may initially be unfamiliar. Paying attention is necessary at all stages of learning—as a pupil, a trainee teacher, and as a working (or non-working) teacher—if you want to keep your practice of the Alexander Technique alive. If you continue paying attention to yourself, you recognise possibilities of other ways of being, as you encounter different experiences of yourself. They may involve a sense of greater integration, or feel like a sort of *expansion*—experiences that can be both universal and unique to you. Having a different experience of yourself may redefine your idea of what is possible: whatever your norm, you are not stuck there; your norm is amenable to change.

There are two implications here. Firstly, you may realise that your internal norm—the way you experience yourself—is not necessarily the way anybody else on the planet experiences themselves. Everybody has their own norm. We each experience ourselves differently from one another. We can't assume that our experiences are the same. Secondly, experiencing yourself differently can help you understand something about your perception and conception of yourself: they relate to your habitual use. In sum, learning the Alexander Technique helps you to see yourself more clearly. Your ground—your way of being, from where you respond to life's stimuli—is somewhat arbitrary. It is based in your use. This ground can be consciously remodelled.

My intention is to get you—whoever you are—to ask yourself some basic questions and to keep asking them:

- Notwithstanding all the improvements to my use since starting to learn and apply the Alexander Technique, is this as good as it gets? Is there room for further improvement?
- Can I refine my practice of the basic principles and continue refining my manner of use?
- What is there about my use that I am unaware of?
- Am I really doing what I think I am doing?

These questions never cease to be relevant. They assume that you don't know everything—you are not omniscient, and you (still) don't know what you don't know. It is okay to keep asking yourself: what don't I know?

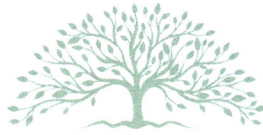

CHAPTER 1

Definitions

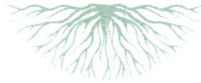

It is worth noting that words and ideas that we may have thought were 'ours' crop up elsewhere. Other disciplines might use the same words but mean something different. Therefore, we need to be clear about the meanings we attach to the words we use.

Explanations of the Alexander Technique sometimes confuse its benefits with the way of getting them and attempts at scientific explanation. In the previous pages, I mention some benefits (the goodies), move on to introductory comments about how we develop them (giving attention to our way of being) and touch on a possible partial definition (the experience of expansion or greater integration, leading to consideration of our use).

Now an attempt at clearer definitions. There are a number of key concepts in the Alexander Technique lexicon, such as use, primary control, inhibition and direction. To have some confidence that we mean the same thing, I want to explain my understanding of these key concepts. Others may wish to add more concepts, for example, non-doing, but the four I mention seem to me to imply or contain the others.

Primary control relationships

There really isn't a primary control as such. It becomes a something in the sphere of relativity.

F. MATTHIAS ALEXANDER[5]

It is easy to infer from the expression 'primary control' that its meaning is explicit, definite and unambiguous. But this is patently not the case. Understandings vary. Here's mine: 'primary control' describes a set of dynamic (constantly changing) relationships between the head, trunk and limbs.[6,7,8]

---

5   See Alexander D. Murray, *Alexander's Way: Frederick Matthias Alexander in His Own Words and in the Words of Those Who Knew Him* (Alexander Technique Center Urbana, 2015), 124.

6   The primary control 'depends upon a certain use of the head and neck in relation to the use of the rest of the body'. F. Matthias Alexander, *The Use of the Self* (Chaterson, 1946), 46.

7   See F. Matthias Alexander, *The Universal Constant in Living* (Chaterson, 1946):

> I discovered that a certain use of the head in relation to the neck, and of the head and neck in relation to the torso and the other parts of the organism, if consciously and continuously employed, ensures, as was shown in my own case, the establishment of a manner of use of the self as a whole which provides the best conditions for raising the standard of the functioning of the various mechanisms, organs, and systems. (6) And 'a particular relativity of the head to the neck and the head and neck to the other parts of the organism' (121).

8   Letter from FM Alexander to Frank Pierce Jones, December 1945: 'We always use the head and neck relationship when explaining to outsiders and find that it works. There really isn't a primary control as such. It becomes a something in the sphere of relativity.' Murray, *Alexander's Way*, 124.

These relationships are informed by ground contact, and postural and balancing processes, and can be monitored through the breath. Ideally, the primary control relationships are characterised by freedom: they are elastic, not rigid; adaptable to the moment, not fixed in time; and responsive to changing needs, attention and intentions. In the traditional formulation, when the primary control relationships are working well, it means that the head is oriented out (forward and up), relative to the back lengthening and widening, and relative to the arms and legs releasing outwards.[9]

Well-organised primary control relationships are character-ised by freedom and responsiveness in the breathing; breathing and movement generally are facilitated. Movement of the limbs or of breathing does not disturb the overall elastic coordination of a well-organised primary control. In other words, when the primary control[10] is working well, not only is the head oriented out, the back lengthening and widening—sometimes referred to as 'staying back in your back'—and arms and legs releasing outwards, but the breathing is also facilitated, allowing freedom and responsiveness to any demand. When we respond via well-organised primary control relationships to any stimulus, inner or outer—for example, moving in space (outer) or having a thought or experiencing an emotion (inner) — we do not disturb this coordinated elasticity. Further, many people report a sort of 'grounded lightness'.

---

9 The wordiness of this description of the primary control relationships is indicative of the challenge of trying to encapsulate an experience in words. See Marjory Barlow and Trevor Allan Davies, *An Examined Life: Marjory Barlow and the Alexander Technique* (Mornum Time Press, 2002), 64, quoting FM: 'it's no good but it's the best...I can do.... It's the nearest I can get in words to the experience you need to have'. Note that directions describe an outcome, not the means of getting it.

10 When I use the singular term 'primary control', it still indicates a set of relationships.

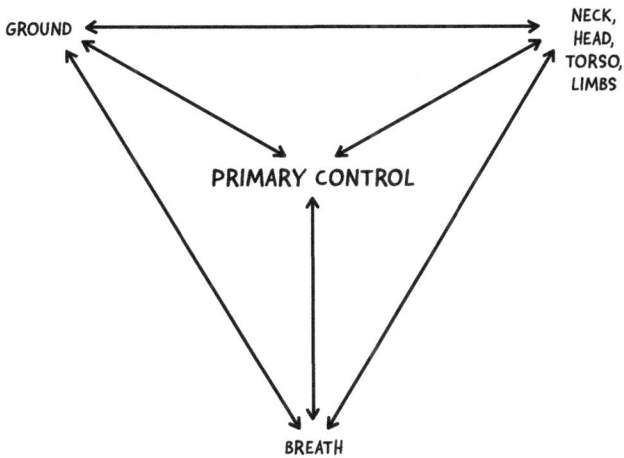

Diagram 1. Each element interacts with all the others

The primary control concept implies that regardless of what else is going on, for example, during movement, thought or emoting, you can work with the idea of consistency in the orientations of relationships. The preferred orientations are defined by freedom and expansion within the relationships between constantly moving parts and external circumstances.[11] The particular 'something in the sphere of relativity' results when you attend to your head/torso/limbs with reference to ground contact and breathing — and one could include more, for example, tongue and jaw — continuously returning to a lively, responsive homeostasis between the moving parts. The primary control is not a switch, a reflex or anything that you can physically point at. It is a set of relationships between things that change.

- Attention to the neck/head/torso/limbs can free the breath and help optimise ground contact.
- Attention to ground contact can inform neck/head/torso/limbs relationships and help optimise the breath.
- Attention to the breath may point to the need to refine neck/head/torso/limbs relationships and quality of ground contact.

All of this has the effect of improving what we refer to as the primary control.

11 See 'Direction: Intent and non-doing', 22.

I suggest that the breathing cannot be fully free and responsive without the particular quality of connected elasticity in the relationships between head, trunk and limbs, which also facilitates the grounded lightness. This is what we recognise as the primary control working well. We don't get grounded lightness without having met the other conditions of positive primary control relationships. Nor do we get it without the breath working freely. When asked how to identify a competent teacher of his Technique, Alexander said that a good teacher could get a pupil breathing better without ever mentioning the breath.[12] This indicates that the teacher has a good understanding of the implicitness of the breath to the conception of the primary control.

Use

You are using your self all the time. You are both the user and the used. The concept of use—having choice in your way of being—implies your ability to influence yourself. Use refers to how you respond to the world: physically (expanding or compressing), emotionally (balanced/intelligently responsive or fearful/overreactive) and mentally (attentive or distracted).[13] None of this is superficial. It is fundamental and defines your way of being. Frank Pierce Jones explained use as 'the total pattern that characterizes a person's responses to

12 See the comment in Robin Simmons' rebuttal of Penelope Easten: Robin Simmons, *The Alexander Technique, Twelve Fundamentals of Integrated Movement—A Critical Review* (Self-published, 2022), 24. It is originally from Catherine 'Kitty' Wielopolska and Marjory Barlow—each made the same comment independently at Stonybrook 1986, heard and relayed by John Nicholls.
13 Note that 'physical', 'emotional' and 'mental' are constructed divisions of our way of being, which is actually simultaneous, continuous and indivisible. If you dig deeply enough, you realise that each division is a facet of the others.

stimuli'.[14] Walter Carrington elegantly said, 'Use indicates the instrumentality of the self in all our dealings with the world.'[15]

The Alexander Technique is a framework for steering your own use of your self—how you respond to what life throws up. The concept of the primary control gives you a measure of your use and a tool to steer it with, so that you can prevent and dismantle acquired maladaptive habits and develop a progressively more integrated level of psycho-physical functioning. Thus, use is anything in the way you respond to life that can potentially come under your conscious control. It is axiomatic that if you are steering, then you want to go in a positive direction. A positive direction means that the way you use your self is oriented towards expansion over time. This indicates a freedom from conditioning which can lead to compression, narrowing or restricting, i.e., blind habit—physically, attentionally or attitudinally.

Inhibition

Creating space between the receipt of a stimulus and your response—and using this space to make a choice about how to proceed and respond to life's various demands, big or small—is inhibition. In this space your system can quieten, in order to make a conscious choice about how you will respond to the situation or event, with reference to your primary control relationships. Then you can go ahead and do what you had intended, do something else or decide to do nothing at all. Inhibition means non-overreactivity. It represents an enlivening opening up of possibilities: allowing time to allow space.

---

14 Frank Pierce Jones, *Freedom to Change: The Development and Science of the Alexander Technique* (Mouritz, 1997), 46.

15 Malcolm Williamson, email to author, July 14, 2024.

Marjory Barlow's formulation of inhibition is 'saying "no" to your first response', to the idea of (doing) something.[16] Inhibition means responding to a stimulus, external or internal, with consideration, as opposed to an immediate reactive response. This allows you time to renew your directions: how am I using my self? It means having a quiet attitude, quiet enough to notice that there is a first response that may include undesirable elements. Then you can choose whether or not to follow this first-response route. Otherwise said, inhibition means giving yourself time to make a choice regarding how to proceed, via reference to the primary control relationships. Walter Carrington used the phrase 'no, not yet... I have time' as an ideal first response, similarly allowing time to refer to the primary control relationships and directions.[17] This is another description of non-reactivity, often also referred to as 'saying "no"' or 'stopping'. Marj Barstow would simply ask, 'What's your hurry?'

We do not inhibit sitting down, standing up, picking up a violin or opening our mouths to speak or sing. We inhibit our first response to the idea of carrying out any of these actions. That is, we check our habitual response to see if we are applying the means that match the result we want, before proceeding. By inhibiting our reactivity, we may discover that we have in fact remained in neutral rather than having already gone down an unconscious, habitual route. Your first response can be 'physical', for example, restricting the breath—a pattern you have repeated until it has become an unconscious habit.

---

16 See, for example, Seán Carey, *Think More, Do Less: Improving Your Teaching and Learning of the Alexander Technique with Marjory Barlow* (HITE, 2017), 48, 60, 79.
17 Walter Carrington, *Thinking Aloud: Talks on Teaching the Alexander Technique* (Mornum Time Press, 1994), 129.

It might be 'emotional'—annoyance, frustration, resentment etc.—which similarly runs along familiar tracks in a predictable pattern. Or else it may be a 'mental' first response—a story you tell yourself—again running a repeated pattern of thoughts, unconscious and now habitual. You want to practise neutral attention: interested and awake yet not reactive; alive and open to our environment yet not overeager; alert but not alarmed. This allows information to arrive before you respond, and without you looking for information. Giving this time allows you to refer back to your primary control relationships. The more you practise inhibition, the more you may notice habitual responses—physical, emotional or mental—which have nothing to do with the actual situation, and to which you can choose to 'withhold consent'.[18] This leaves you freer to make non-habitual choices as you carry out your activity or response.

During my teacher training, a fellow trainee became frustrated with the Alexandrian idea of inhibition as 'stopping'. I think he had fallen into a not-uncommon misunderstanding of inhibition as a deadening non-response, rather than an active process of consciously choosing a course, having inhibited his first response in order to renew his primary control directions, and then proceeding. This common mistake is a mere lip-service 'stop' which doesn't quieten the system at all. The important thing is not the pausing, but the quality of quietening. We want to be quiet enough to allow ourselves

---

18 See Alexander, *Universal Constant*, 107. For example,

> it is an act of inhibition which comes into play when, for instance, in response to a given stimulus, we refuse to give consent to certain activity, and thus prevent ourselves from sending those messages which would ordinarily bring about the habitual reaction resulting in the 'doing' within the self of what we no longer wish to 'do'.

to receive information fully and attentively, to give ourselves time to let go of any anticipatory fixing or presetting, before we start to respond. This quality of initial non-reactivity most observably extends to the physical. But it may also include emotional and mental elements. FM Alexander also referred to the 'spiritual'.[19] We want to be receptive, yet non-reactive, to all the things we don't yet know about as well as the ones we do. This is the meaning of FM's inhibition.

If we reason that the familiar needs changing, not doing a physical action means not doing it in the old, familiar way. This does not mean suppressing, nor overriding it, for example, imposing a particular body position over the top of something that already constitutes an unnecessary 'doing'. Indeed, overriding the old habit is an extra 'doing'. We rather need to catch the habitual response before it takes hold. This means truly staying in neutral, open or available to new possibilities, that is, remaining uncommitted to how you will reach your goal other than by working with reference to your primary control relationships. This is being non-reactive while remaining awake, attentive, receptive and responsive. An example: you are going home at the end of your working day. You plan to pick up groceries on the way. Suddenly, you arrive at home and then remember that you needed to go via the shops. Yet here you are at home, without groceries. You had been on autopilot and simply followed your well-rehearsed route home. To have gone via the shops would have required that you stay alert at the critical junction, where you had to not go left, but rather turn right. The two possibilities are mutually exclusive. Not going left allows for fulfilling the aspiration of going right. Without not left, there would be no possibility of going right.

19 'You translate everything, whether physical, mental or spiritual, into muscular tension.' F. Matthias Alexander, *Aphorisms* (Mouritz, 2000), 36.

In a similar way, without not tightening the neck, there is no possibility of lengthening.

With an emotional response, it's not that we don't want to feel or express emotion. But the emotion is ideally an authentic response to the present conditions. It is not just 'how I always react', an unconsidered pattern which may have all sorts of unwanted or unconsidered ramifications.

With our thoughts, do we really need to cycle through that retelling of a story that justifies a habitual behaviour or attitude? An example of habitual storytelling: imagine looking out through a window and seeing a tree. You recognise that it is a tree. You might even know what sort of tree it is. It may evoke memories—arguments about where to plant it, whether to chop it down or whose responsibility it is. However, at this point, you are looking through the window and simply seeing the tree. You can recognise the tree neutrally, while maintaining your physical distance from it. You do not need to go out and smell the tree, feel its bark or give it a hug. You can maintain your distance, allow the visual information to arrive to you and perceive 'tree', i.e., you can dispassionately observe, perhaps remembering, but without needing to rerun old stories or judgements. This principle is vital when experiencing unfamiliar sensations. You don't want to follow or examine a new sensation, but rather observe it dispassionately.

Importantly, to control a pattern of behaviour, i.e., to move from the habitual to the conscious, the inhibition of your first response to something needs to continue and be continuous throughout the ensuing action. Inhibition means maintaining neutrality and responsiveness, not getting invested in the outcome at the 'critical moment'[20] (gaining your end in

---

20 Alexander, *Use of the Self*, 10.

your usual way), and maintaining your positive conditions of use with reference to the primary control relationships throughout what ensues. To take the mundane, yet instructive, example of coming to standing from sitting: on framing an intention to stand, and deciding to move, you first remember to exercise your inhibitory intention to not tighten your neck, pull your head back, shorten your back or to tense your legs (or whatever variations of these words you use). You then need to continuously reaffirm these decisions throughout the action of standing and beyond. That is, inhibition applies both before and during the movement. In fact, you want no discontinuity between before, during or after. With a too-quick reaction, you are likely already locked in, committed to your usual response. The potential for choice, allowing for something different, is lost; your quality of balance may also be lost, along with your physical neutrality. Balance or detachment allow responsiveness. You want to remain as close as possible to being a 'blank canvas' for as long as possible. This means remaining neutral and not preset at any level in the way you respond. It is a sort of attitudinally non-invested way of being.

Inhibition and sensation

An initial encounter with the Alexander Technique often results in a striking new experience of oneself. This is an example of an 'internal input'. We want to repeat it—we think, 'This feels good,' and then risk following the feeling into the body. But the observation that it feels good should remain just that: an observation. The instant we follow it, it is no longer a dispassionate observation, but becomes a 'doing' with its associated 'feeling'—feeling something out. The focus shifts from a neutral, observational stance to something that includes judgement, that seeks to name, identify or feel something, whether expected and familiar, or novel and unfamiliar.

All of these are kinds of doing. Of course, sensation of any sort is liable to draw our attention. For example, pain can take over our attention completely, so that we focus only on the pain and lose our ability to influence the things we are capable of influencing. Our response to pain may narrow our attention, taking it away from the pain's broader context. However, we are capable of recognising sensation without descending into it. In fact, we are constantly receiving sensory information about our internal and external environments. With practice, we become capable of observing this with non-attachment. This is the meaning of 'leaving yourself alone'.[21] The habit of wanting to explore sensation is not detached observation but rather an involved 'rummaging'.[22,23] This invariably leads to a loss of liveliness and responsiveness. By applying inhibition, we can 'say no' to following sensation and rather experience it without trying to feel it out—we can maintain detachment. The new sensation can simply prompt neutral interest, but not attachment. We can choose not to be diverted into fascination with an effect, but to stick to renewal of our means-oriented path of inhibition and direction.

Realistically, these ideas represent an aspiration. We are always being distracted by goals and attachments or self-judgements. A distraction is anything that pulls us away from neutral receptivity. We are more likely to achieve our goal without unnecessary effort when we let go of attachment to

---

21 Carrington, *Thinking Aloud*, 58, 71.
22 Marjory Barlow said that we must not 'do' our directions 'even a teeny-weeny bit'. Barlow and Davies, *Examined Life*, 130.
23 See Carrington, *Thinking Aloud*, 62:
> They wish the up to happen, but since they don't really set much store on the wish, they will just do it a little bit, just to make sure, just to be on the safe side, they'll introduce just a little bit of doing.

In other words, we don't really trust that thinking is enough and that we all very subtly do something to get the 'up'.

its achievement or to judging how well we are doing, i.e., by applying inhibition. As we pay attention to ourselves, we may realise that we keep diverging from neutral. Ideally, we then quietly let go of such distractions, over and over again.[24]

In summary, inhibition—responding without physically compressing nor mentally or emotionally fixing—means

1. Stopping to give time to make a choice: being open, awake, attentive, alive and receptive to information, internal or external, yet not reactive to it. It involves cultivating a light, effortless quality of attention (to both inside and outside, i.e., self and environment); and

2. Continuing our non-reactive attention/intention at the critical moment of giving consent to proceed—continuously not going the way we have reasoned that we wish to avoid, as we allow the 'right' thing to happen.

Direction: Intent and non-doing

When an investigation comes to be made, it will be found that
every single thing we are doing in the Work is exactly what
is being done in nature where the conditions are right, the
difference being that we are learning to do it consciously.

F. MATTHIAS ALEXANDER[25]

If Alexander's primary control resides in relationships, then directions are an attempt to describe desirable orientations within these constantly changing relationships. The directions bring life, energy and intent to these relationships (between

---

24 Note the difference between attention and awareness. Paying attention is an active state of curious interest, which may lead to increasing awareness. Awareness is an effect; attention is the means.

25 Alexander, *Aphorisms*, 88.

head, trunk and limbs) and bespeak a quality of coherent aliveness or springy elasticity. There is an energetic flow to direction, a fluency which is malleable and definitely not stiff. It is a process of 'wishing and willing'[26] what you want to have happen, which may involve something like visualisation, and includes a dynamic relationing in the body, sometimes called oppositional or antagonistic pulls.[27] Direction has a lively intent that includes an aspect of 'body', yet without attachment to 'body'. Directions mean inhabiting the body with detached intent and awakeness.[28] This does not require sensation.

Poor use in a person can often be seen in an awkward agglomeration of tightening, including in the neck and elsewhere; shortening, compromising freedom of the breath and quality of ground contact, along with a reactivity that does not recognise these conditions and their influence.[29] Hence the need for the typical directions, preceded by inhibition of the habitual.

The directions represent an expression of intent. The words describing how we want our primary control relationships give us an expression of our directional aspiration.[30] The intent is to steer, improve and refine the relationships between

---

26 See Carrington, *Thinking Aloud*, 15.

27 I use 'oppositional' to include 'antagonistic'.

28 See the footnote on direction in Alexander, *Use of the Self*, 13: '[C]onducting...energy to the...mechanisms.'

29 For instance, any undue tension in the legs affects all coordination. See detail regarding legs (in Chapter 4: 'General specifics and practical explorations') under 'Semi-flexion', page 59, and Explorations 1–8.

30 Classic words for the directions are 'allow the neck to be free, to allow the head to go forward and up, to allow the back to lengthen and widen, and the knees to go forward and away'. Other forms of words, for example, 'let the head lead and the body follow', are also perfectly valid and can also be unpacked to extract the meaning.

the elements of the primary control, resulting in overall integration and expansion. Directions remind us that we are using our selves and that we can direct this use. They also give us a helpful form of words to frame our intent. When we direct, we are more or less formally giving attention to ourselves. The content of the directions summarises how we wish to organise ourselves. The directions are a way of making conscious and deliberate the process of undoing what we don't want, and remembering what we do want. If we have some idea of our primary control relationships, we can explore and work on ourselves using our directions. Directions have an enlivening or waking-up effect. With direction, we inhabit ourselves more fully and deeply. In using our directions, we bring ourselves back to that most immediate touchstone or reference point: that of our body. The story of AR Alexander's accident illustrates this. FM's brother, AR Alexander, suffered a catastrophic spinal injury. Doctors told him he would never walk again. But lying for months in bed, he worked patiently with his directions and was eventually able to walk, albeit with an unusual gait.[31]

Why direct?

In 1910, Alexander wrote that we cannot rely on instinct to adapt successfully to all the new, fast-changing technologies of modern living.[32] The level of general stimulation that we

---

31 This anecdote may be a little simplistic or apocryphal. See Frank Pierce Jones, *Body Awareness in Action: Study of the Alexander Technique* (Schocken, 1976), 69. Jones describes AR Alexander and his recovery after the horse-riding accident which smashed his spine. AR's daily walk took him to the park, where a passer-by commented to AR, seated on a park bench, 'Sir, I've watched you for a long time and I wish I knew what you have that other people don't have.'

32 F. Matthias Alexander, *Man's Supreme Inheritance* (Chaterson, 1946), 143: 'Whilst under the guidance of the subconscious mind, mankind cannot readily adapt itself to the rapidly and ever-changing conditions imposed by civilization.'

are subject to has certainly not decreased since then. Without direction, our use tends to deteriorate because of our tendency to end-gain: in the face of overstimulation, and relying on 'instinct', we try to achieve our goals without first making sure we have the necessary and sufficient means to achieve them.[33] Think of this as being like entropy, a gradual decline into disorder: without direction we tend to become ever more out of balance. If we react without forethought, i.e., without inhibition and reference to our directions, chances are that our reactions will involve compression at some level. If we continue that way, we end up using our selves worse than if we stop and think about how to respond. As we age, there is in any case a loss of elasticity in our tissues. Even if we were just minimally active in a low-stimulus environment, yet without direction, I believe that over time there would arise a sort of non-responsive, poor quality of tone. Direction maintains a degree of liveliness.

When we first start learning the Alexander Technique, we typically think the directions linearly, in words—we start with one direction, add another, then maybe a third or fourth.[34] That is, they start by being entirely sequential—one after another. The longer we work with them in this sequential way,

---

33 There are undoubtedly individuals who use themselves well. Fred Astaire is often cited as an example, as more recently is Roger Federer. But do they sufficiently understand themselves to be able to maintain their good use in the face of some disruption to it? Alexander not only articulated the concept of use and how to steer it, but also devised a way of communicating about it using his hands.

34 It is worth noting that with any direction, for example, 'head forward and up', you must consider what it is in relation to. What is the *context* for the neck to be free? Head forward and up *in relation to what*? Back back in relation to what? Knees forward and away in relation to what? The answers might vary slightly between individuals, depending on their conditions and manner of use.

the more continuous they become—instead of occurring one after another, they start to blend together. We need to become skilled at juggling these many thoughts, one after another, all together.[35] At some point, well along in our practice, our mental process might become more of a continuous checklist and it may or may not be word-based. We might get to a stage where, almost instantaneously, as we start with the neck, the whole cascade of directions is triggered, even as we simultaneously go through them one at a time ('Neurons that fire together wire together').[36] Getting to this point undoubtedly requires consistency and repetition, i.e., discipline in attentiveness to ourselves. Our attention needs to remain mobile, as we lightly loop through our directions more or less continuously. Directions could be imagined as travelling along particular neural message pathways: we build these through practice such that they become easier to access; our intent permeates our being, extending to the cells of our extremities; and the message pathways link up into an internal web of awakeness, an internet of integrated, informed being, or background of intent.

Objections to directing and inhibiting

I believe that objections to directing are usually based on erroneous preconceptions or learned misconceptions. The word 'direction' can be interpreted such that directions become stiff and do-y. During my training, a teacher visiting the training course observed our class practising semi-flexion and putting hands on the back of a chair, and commented that we looked like a bunch of stiff, frightened rabbits. That suggests to me that perhaps we were not directing as I now understand it—and happily my current concept of directing is not stuck in

---

35 Alexander, *Use of the Self*, 20.
36 See "Hebb's Law," in Donald Hebb, *The Organisation of Behaviour: A Neuropsychological Theory* (John Wiley & Sons, 1949).

that early experience. That is, I do not associate this frightened-rabbit mode of application with the word 'direction'.

I have spoken to some teachers who claim not to direct. I assume they mean that they direct differently to how they originally understood directing. Similarly, some teachers find 'inhibition' problematic. This also often represents an issue with the meaning that they have attached to these words. They seem to have learnt that inhibition is an awkward, obstinate refusal to act and that direction is an (over)doing. When these misunderstood versions of inhibition and direction are combined, there is an overall stiffness rather than neutral responsiveness.

Not 'doing' the directions

Here is an analogy for the process of directing: imagine an old-fashioned factory floor, where some item is manufactured. It is a complex process that involves various components, each of which has to be worked on before ultimately being put together as the finished item. Many people are involved in the process of completing the item. The factory owner sits in their glass-panelled mezzanine office, where they have an overview, from where they can issue directives, while watching what happens on the floor. They are clear that their job is to remain in the control centre. It is not their job to do any of the actual labour. Their job is to work out what needs to happen, seeing how each element of the process relates to the other elements, and to issue orders. They communicate what it is that they want done, and let their staff get on with it. They do not do anything themselves. Thus it is with directing: clarity of intent remains key. Direction resides at the level of intent, and intent must not become doing. The factory owner, representing your intent and vision of what is wanted, directs. The trustworthy staff—your nervous system—carries out the owner's intent. The owner doesn't check on them. Anything else would constitute interference. Rummaging, for instance, describes trying to feel out direction, and this is a doing.[37]

If you were learning to direct from a book, you would likely fall into all the potential pitfalls. Alexander describes these in *The Use of the Self*.[38] Actually, I suspect that all of us manage to fall into all the potential pitfalls even when learning from a teacher, but a teacher can usually help us past them much more quickly than we can manage on our own. Indeed, the pitfalls are part of the learning process. Arguably, they are the learning process—we experience and identify problems, and get distance and perspective by working through our own perceptual and conceptual mistakes. This deepens our practice. And it recurs repeatedly.

37 Regarding 'feeling directions out', see the reference to rummaging under 'Inhibition and sensation', page 21.
38 See "Chapter 1," in Alexander, *Use of the Self*, 6–24.

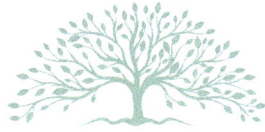

CHAPTER 2

Teacher training and the Alexander Technique journey

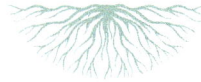

A structured process of working on yourself—what you get in a training programme over sufficient time—gives you key teaching skills. There are different training models, but a three-year teacher-training plan may look roughly like this: the first year generally aims at trainees being able to work on themselves effectively and reliably. In the second year, the level of demand goes up, as trainees work on each other under supervision. They learn to maintain their own positive manner of use while dealing with the added stimulus of putting their hands on somebody else. In the third year, trainees learn to apply all of the foregoing to a real teaching situation, as they also give verbal instructions. All the while, the trainee continues to work on their own use of themselves.

The process of training to teach the Alexander Technique is an intensive, deeper and more precise version of the self-work learnt in regular lessons. Improving your use depends on you applying the principles of inhibition and direction, and gradually deepening your understanding of those principles, both kinaesthetically and intellectually. Through applying inhibition and direction to traditional procedures and general activities, you learn teaching skills. This relates most obviously to hands-on skills. With the support of your trainer, you sustain deeper inhibition, even more than you think you are capable of; you learn more about the power of inhibition and direction, and your capacity to carry them through. These experiences are also valuable when taken into non-hands-on elements of teaching.

In most traditions of Alexander Technique teaching, touch and words are the two main modalities of instruction. When a teacher uses their hands in teaching, the obvious thing to notice is that they touch their pupil—this is an 'outer practice'. It looks straightforward but there is a great deal that is unseen, implicit and experiential. It is this unseen, inner content that is important and key to effective communication. If we want to teach well, effective communication is vital. The quality of the outer practice rests completely on the quality of performance of the inner practice: the practice of inhibition and direction.[39]

A structured process should scaffold working on your use and learning the effective use of your hands, i.e., in a way that integrates both you and whomever you touch when teaching. Discipline is needed to develop confidence in working with a means-oriented approach using the principles of inhibition and direction. Whatever words we use to describe Alexander's principles and whatever shiny new reframing we come up with, the twin skills of inhibition and direction provide a necessary foundation for personal evolution and for developing teaching

---

39 See 'Inhibition', page 15; and 'Direction: Intent and non-doing', page 22.

skills. These are the skills we teach. A natural outcome of learning to apply inhibition and direction to ourselves, as we engage with using our hands, is hands that can communicate effectively. In all this, effective and supportive feedback from trainer to trainee is vital.[40] A carefully structured teacher training should offer this discipline and the ensuing confidence in the use of the hands. Cultivating an effectively directed, non-doing way of using your hands obliges you to engage with inhibition and direction. There is no escape. You stand a better chance of developing higher-level skills if you keep aiming at refining your hands-on skills.

In addition to hand contact, the verbal component of teaching is crucial. The discipline and principles involved in learning to use our hands apply to the multiple other teaching skills, for example, what we say and how we say it. Words can convey relevant information at the right moment, as the teacher coordinates and complements information from their hands with explanation, encouragement, support, commentary, relationship-building, or an anecdote or other story. And sometimes silence is the best communication.

Whether you are the learner or the teacher, the emphasis is always on process, not outcome. You, as trainee, and later as teacher, work on whatever you can steer in this moment—your manner of use—optimising what is available right now.[41] You learn to understand the practical reality of the concepts of the Alexander Technique—use, primary control, inhibition and direction—and the connections between them. Whether you are a trainee or a teacher, as you gradually deepen your understanding of the practical meaning of the concepts

40 See 'Why traditional procedures?', page 44.
41 See "Chapter 1," in Alexander, *Universal Constant*, 1–11.

offered in words, you internalise them. You progressively embody the concepts. Before we can hope to teach anyone the Alexander Technique, we need to exemplify what we want to teach, through our own practice and application of it. We need to have gone through the process of cultivating how to work effectively on ourselves. Beyond the end of formal teacher training, we continue the learning process by living the open-ended nature of that learning.[42]

Learning and teaching inhibition and direction

Inhibition involves non-overreactivity, allowing an alert, neutral, open quietness, a responsiveness which is detached from expectations or the need for particular outcomes. Inhibition allows for the possibility of new outcomes. Upon this rests our ability for direction—energised intent without doing. The more we can cultivate our alert-yet-detached quietness, the more effective our direction can be. This is a meaning of 'non-doing'. We don't help direction along with little 'degrees of doing', but rather leave ourselves alone.[43,44,45]

---

42 For example, see FM Alexander quoted in Goddard Binkley, *The Expanding Self* (STAT Books, 1993), 51:
   Why, Mr. Binkley, when I am teaching you, as I do now, I am able to convey to you what I want to convey, because as I touch you, and guide you with my hands in carrying out my instructions, I, myself, am going up! up! up!
43 Carrington, *Thinking Aloud*, 58, 62, 71.
44 See Nanette Walsh, "Peggy Williams in Her Own Words," *AmSAT News*, no. 63 (2004): 19.
45 See 'Inhibition', page 15; and 'Direction: Intent and non-doing', page 22.

In lessons with private pupils, the teacher might use a variety of activities to convey what inhibition and direction mean in practice. In traditional teacher-training courses, the outer practice may be refined and generalised to various procedures (for example, hands on the back of a chair or whispered ahs), which can become a laboratory for all the abstract inner processes. These procedures encapsulate what we need to learn and develop: our capacity to meet a demand with expanding use (also referred to as oppositional pulls), via inhibition and direction.

Touch

In a sense, teaching the Alexander Technique has very little to do directly with our hands. They are a medium for conveying a range of information. Our hands are emphatically not used as in other fields, for example, massage, physiotherapy, osteopathy or chiropractic. In the Alexander Technique, your hands are the extremities of an integrated system, which includes your head, your feet and how they touch the ground, and everything in between including the function of your breathing. How well your hands work—their sensitivity and responsiveness—depends entirely on how well coordinated and integrated your system is. In other words, it's the use of your self, not merely the use of your hands, that affects your pupil. The quality of your touch is a function of your entire body, informed by the clarity of your thinking. This develops with time.[46]

---

46 See 'Direction: Intent and non-doing', page 22; 'Why hands?', page 40; and 'Practising', page 106.

We use our hands all the time in living: to reach, pick up, hold and manipulate (anything). The habitual use of our hands is deeply ingrained. You can appear to have good understanding of your use in general, yet as soon as your hands come into play when teaching, the quality of your use can diminish. But this is not a reason for hands-off teaching: quite the reverse. It should be a spur to refine your hands-on skills. Cultivating the discipline of inhibition and direction, when applied to something as deeply habitual as using your hands, helps you build confidence both in applying inhibition and direction, as well as through the positive outcome of their application.

Training strengths and weaknesses, and working with them

During the time it takes to reach a beginning-teacher level, you ideally immerse yourself not only in the practice of the Alexander Technique, but also in the relevant history, literature, physiology and anatomy, pedagogy, science and so on. This immersion is the beginning—what you do with what you learn depends on you. Your training course sets a tone, expectation, ethos, context and aspiration, and provides a model. Yet training courses are different from one another—they assume different things, they have their own ethos, attitudes, beliefs and emphases, subtle and not so subtle, some overt and others unspoken. The head of training promulgates their own strengths and weaknesses and areas of interest. All trainers have blind spots—things that they take for granted, assume and believe. It can't be otherwise. Thus, there are potential pitfalls and positives in any training approach.

Communication can fail due to either the teacher or the trainee. Teachers, including trainers, get misunderstood, they may miscommunicate their message and messages can get filtered through trainees' own preconceptions. Trainees do not always 'hear' what is said to them in the way it was meant or do not accurately register at a kinaesthetic level what has happened. Their focus of attention or expectations may not match their teacher's. Different individuals take different insights and interpretations from the same teachers. Some trainees hear everything uncritically, others question everything, ideally without attachment to any biases. We still pander to our habits. The choices we make may leave out potentially useful learnings—we might miss opportunities to deepen or broaden particular elements of our learning.

The Alexander Technique can be transformational, and during the intensity of teacher training, this may be particularly so. But attachment to how or what you learnt during training—how it was taught or what you understood—can be a stumbling block to further development. It is important to remain open to a continuing evolution of understanding, for example, of key concepts like primary control, inhibition and direction, or of hands-on skills. Having the humility to realise that there may be a difference between what was taught and what was learnt may be helpful. The more we think deeply about our skills and their basis in understanding and beliefs, the more we can develop as teachers. We need to remain students as well as teachers. Once qualified, the cultivation of all our teaching skills can be ongoing. The transition into ever-greater competence can continue.

Use your superpower!

Teacher Rachel Zahn brought the Alexander Technique world's attention to the work of Francisco Varela.[47] A late-twentieth century scientist, he recognised the problematic nature of dualistic mind–body thinking, somewhat as FM Alexander did one hundred years earlier. There is a difference between first-person experience (our internal experience of an event or of ourselves) and third-person experience (that of a detached observer, for example, a physiotherapist). A well-trained, competent Alexander Technique teacher can provide a second-person viewpoint. The Alexander teacher has the capacity to act as an intermediary between first-person experience and third-person 'objectivity'. Via their specially trained hands-on skills, the Alexander teacher can perceive potentially significant information about their pupil, which the pupil is often not aware of. Simultaneously the teacher can convey to the pupil relevant deep information through their hands. These dual hands-on skills of perception and conveyance are what make Alexander Technique teachers unique. Alexander teachers shouldn't hesitate to use and continue to develop these special skills.[48]

What is our job as Alexander Technique teachers?

The job of a good Alexander teacher is to help their pupils learn how to work on themselves effectively and to apply this work to the art of living. The teacher helps their pupils

47 See, for example, Francisco J. Varela and Jonathan Shear, "First-person Methodologies: What, Why, How?" *Journal of Consciousness Studies* 6, nos. 2–3 (1999): 1–14.
48 See 'Online teaching', page 149.

experience their primary control relationships working better and to understand how to steer this for themselves. This is synonymous with offering an experience of integration, including improvement in breathing, balance, movement and potentially other aspects, for example, emotional. A good teacher complements the use of their hands with relevant verbal information, clearly articulating the what, how and why, and can help their pupil understand and connect these.

Some teachers describe their work in terms of helping their pupil recognise and change poor habits (of use). Learning to apply inhibition and direction allows the pupil access to constructive change. The poor habits we want to recognise are those that render our primary control relationships less effective than they could be and, therefore, lower our general standard of functioning. Why put this process in terms of the primary control, inhibition and direction?[49] There is a danger in not being clear about the depth and extent of the influence of the primary control relationships, and how to work on them. For example, the goal can easily be reduced and limited to 'ease of movement'. However, Alexander recognised that the concept of a primary control is central, and it provides a route to steering our use—the 'universal constant in living'. 'Use' is a sort of meta-concept, a general tool. It acknowledges the instrumentality of the self. To develop a way of working with the primary control—a set of dynamic relationships between parts of the self—the teacher may bring the pupil's attention to anything that gets in the way of deeper integration

---

49 See Alexander, *Universal Constant*, 6–7:
>   I had found a way by which we can judge whether the influence of our manner of use is affecting our general functioning adversely or otherwise, the criterion being whether or not this manner of use is interfering with the correct employment of the primary control.

of these parts. Superficially, this might be some unconsciously imposed, habitual pattern of physical tension. Less superficially, this might lead to a consideration of the breath.[50] Underneath that might lie attitudes, beliefs, biases or misconceptions that determine our assumptions. Teaching the Alexander Technique comes back to conveying inhibition and direction, however you name them—a non-reactive energisation—as a way of working on oneself, to learn the 'control of human reaction'.[51]

---

50 Crucially, Alexander recognised that 'all physical effort tends to increase thoracic rigidity and to cause breathlessness'. Alexander, *Universal Constant*, 43.
51 See Alexander, *Use of the Self*, 26, 28, 54.

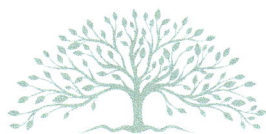

CHAPTER 3

Hands, traditional procedures and time

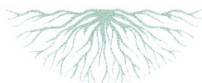

In order to communicate his work, FM Alexander began using his hands early in his teaching career.[52] He progressively developed his manual skills over his lifetime, and those who knew him reported that his skills reached a peak in his last years, notwithstanding that he suffered a stroke in 1949. Developing skill in hands-on work is not easy, but rather demands rigorous initial guidance in, and ongoing application of, inhibition and direction. Traditional procedures provide a wonderful vehicle for this endeavour. And time spent on these during formal training and after is repaid in gains in proficiency and depth of understanding.

As time goes on, there are fewer Alexander Technique teachers who learnt from first-generation teachers. Some aspects of teaching and learning that were earlier considered

---

52 See, for example, Barlow and Davies, *Examined Life*, 65.

fundamental and non-negotiable have consequently tended to become more optional. Their depth and value are not always appreciated. The particular use of the hands needed in teaching the Alexander Technique, in order to effectively communicate inhibition and direction, requires time and careful attention to cultivate, which are returned in skill and understanding. We should remain curious about why first-generation teachers worked the way they did.

Why hands?

The hands are the most convenient part of the anatomy with which to touch. They can touch with extraordinary sensitivity. Even for someone who has not trained to use their hands in an Alexandrian way, the hands' sensitivity is orders of magnitude greater than that in most other parts of the body. Plus, the hands have a convenient 'delivery system', the arms, that enable us to get them wherever we want. In teaching the Alexander Technique, a particular quality of hand contact is desirable. It can be described as soft yet firm; elastic yet guiding; both giving and accepting, and perhaps other pairings.

Hands can convey inhibition

> We put our hands on a pupil to gather information, not to do something to them. We do not take our pupil up; we help them to recognise when they are pulling down and to be able to stop doing it.
>
> WALTER CARRINGTON[53]

The hands can convey calm and quiet. The more the teacher has embodied a quality of deep, non-reactive quiet, i.e., inhibition, the more their hands can convey this, and the

---

53 He said this in class on various occasions.

more the pupil has the opportunity to recognise this quality as a possibility for themselves. It is this quality of neutral 'being there yet not needing to do anything' that underlies the communication through our hands. Communication means information both from and to the pupil. Quiet, non-doing hands allow the teacher to 'listen' to their pupil. The hands are a conduit for the pupil to the teacher's own inner quality of non-doing, non-judgemental, accepting, quiet openness. Through their hands, the teacher talks to their pupil's whole nervous system, including their brain, asking for 'quiet', which may then allow direction to be cultivated. That is, the teacher's hands help to quieten habitual messages between the pupil's brain and muscles—they support inhibition. This allows for the possibility of something else to happen: direction becomes more available.

Hands gather information about relationships of parts

The hands can inform the teacher about their pupil's conditions and manner of use via the pupil's primary control relationships—up, down, fixed (to what extent and where), collapsed, elastic, integrated, with breathing that involves balanced tone—and where the interrelationships might become freer. I recall a particular lesson early on in my Alexander Technique life. My teacher, Tessa Cawdron, had her hands on my neck and head. From there she pointed out to me that I was stiffening my ankles. She was of course right, and I was stunned. How she knew seemed mysterious to me then, but is perfectly clear now.

A well-trained teacher's hands can instantly bring the teacher a wealth of information, including about parts other than the ones their hands are touching. This is because of the relationships between all the parts. For example, if the pupil locks their knees, a pattern of adjustments that is characteristic of locked knees is triggered to maintain balance in the body. Thus, the pupil does not just lock their knees, but also tightens in their lower back, restricts their rib movement in a particular way and creates a downward drag all the way to the head, all linked back to the knees. It is an interdependent pattern.

It is worth noting that we simply do not know, a priori, what an individual's 'optimal' relationship of spinal curves might look like. This is dependent on the context of the individual's use in general; this information can come through the teacher's hands.

Hands and the pupil's quality of attention

Again, the hands can inform the teacher about the pupil's quality of attention and the clarity of their directing. The hands potentially receive immediate feedback about the pupil's responsiveness — the teacher may be able to tell if the pupil is daydreaming (referred to as 'drift' in Irene Tasker's notes),[54] overdoing or trying to feel something out. Thus, the hands can help inform the teacher's verbal instructions and feedback to the pupil.[55]

Hands and words

You see the purpose of the hands is to put meaning into those words, those directions that you're teaching them to give.

MARJORY BARLOW[56]

---

54 Regina Stratil, *Irene Tasker: Her Life and Work with the Alexander Technique* (Mouritz, 2020), 258.
55 See 'Direction: Intent and non-doing', page 22.
56 See Barlow and Davies, *Examined Life*, 64.

Using their hands, the teacher can confirm whether their pupil is getting the desired message, or not.[57] They can offer immediate feedback: no, not *that*, but *this*. Their hands can also clarify their use of words and what they mean by the words, for example, helping to bring precise meaning to words like 'neck free' and other phrases that they use. This allows the pupil to build their own conceptual framework upon which to hang their experiences. Conversely, the hands can hint to the teacher what might be usefully conveyed verbally to their pupil to move things on conceptually, to help the pupil towards greater free integration. Hands and words together help the pupil marry and make sense of their perceptions (what they feel) and their conceptions (how they understand what they feel).

FM's hands

At times, FM Alexander was famously wanting in his verbal explanations. However, he had extraordinary manual skills. The short video of FM working[58] was filmed after he had been developing his skill for over fifty years. Watching it, one is struck by the way he positions his hands—one on the pupil's head, the other on their upper back. He appears to be constantly playing one hand off against the other, managing a deep, dynamic interplay between them and what they tell him, as well as what they are able to impart to the pupil in the moment. FM clearly gets the pupil's head going forward and up, and their back lengthening and widening.[59] Most of us teachers don't have the skill to do this in the way FM demonstrates.

---

57 See 'Hands', page 118.
58 "FM Alexander Film narrated by Walter Carrington," film, posted September 27, 2024, YouTube, 7:20, https://www.youtube.com/watch?v=Bz3a0EJKDIs.
59 People who had lessons with FM reported that it felt like his top hand was 'sucking them upwards'. John Nicholls quotes Dilys Carrington on this.

A careful consideration of the relationships of the pupil's cervical, thoracic and lumbar curves may suggest more. It looks as if FM is constantly listening with his hands and feeding back about these relationships, in a non-verbal conversation with the pupil.[60] FM's lower hand could be monitoring the pupil's thoracic curve, and its relationship to their cervical curve. His upper hand may be communicating with the pupil's thoracic area about the head and neck and their relationship, and vice versa. An understanding of these curves and their relationships may be another way of understanding 'forward and up'.[61] Indeed, forward and up is not necessarily confined to the relationship between neck and head.

Why traditional procedures?

The placing of the pupil in what would ordinarily be considered an abnormal position (of mechanical advantage) affords the teacher an opportunity to establish the mental and physical guiding principles which enable the pupil after a short time to repeat the coordination with the same perfection in a normal position.

F. MATTHIAS ALEXANDER[62]

Using drills such as scales and arpeggios, a musician achieves technical mastery of their instrument so that clarity of musical expression is available to them. Similarly, traditional Alexander Technique procedures are a route towards mastery of our own instrument: the self and how to act through it. This mastery includes when we use our hands in teaching, such that

60 See, for example, Stratil, *Irene Tasker*: 'necessity of two hands working in coordination' (254) and 'FM's hands are always working relatively to one another' (260).
61 I am indebted to Joan Murray, Merran Poplar, Luc Vanier and Rebecca Nettl-Fiol for this insight.
62 Alexander, *Man's Supreme Inheritance*, 115.

anything we do is underpinned by elastic expansion. Traditional procedures are the scales and arpeggios of Alexander Technique teacher training. That is why they are typically used on teacher-training courses. Like scales in music, traditional procedures strip the Alexander Technique to the essentials. They provide a structured form within which to recognise, practise, refine and reflect on the basics: the application of inhibition and direction to a given situation, with the aim of learning to respond to a demand with coordinated elasticity. Effectively practising traditional procedures also results in improving our use. Procedures formalise an abstract framework, one more detached than a conventional activity is from a recognisable outcome. Traditional procedures can provide us with a way of working on ourselves well beyond the end of formal training, and may be included when swapping work with other teachers.

Traditional procedures allow us to externalise what is an internal process. They provide a template which can be applied to anything: 'guiding principles which enable...the same perfection in a normal position'.[63] That is, you use them in working on optimising primary control relationships. With traditional procedures you work within constraints so that you have only the use of your self to focus on. Yet the procedures are 'not a perimeter but an aperture: a space through which the world... [can be] seen'.[64] As in any creative process, having constraints obliges us to look more deeply at what remains available and what we can do with it. The constraints created by the 'rules' (the boundaries of form) of the traditional

63 Alexander, *Man's Supreme Inheritance*, 115. I suggest that 'guiding principles' refers to the recognition and activation of the primary control relationships.
64 Robert Macfarlane, "Introduction," in Shepherd, *Living Mountain*.

procedures can invite curiosity and creativity, resulting in greater depth of understanding. They ask us to delve into meaning and significance in a way we tend not to when we have an unlimited choice. Constraints make us think more carefully about our choices and where they can lead us. Working on ourselves in daily life, without boundaries, without form in the sense of kata,[65] makes it more difficult to see relationships and build as much out of our practice. The purpose of a traditional procedure is no more and no less than that of carrying out the procedure with inhibition and direction: ultimate application. The procedures are not attached to an external goal but are rather about practising means, developing oppositional elasticity as a way of being.

Thus, traditional procedures give us a structure for the practice of discipline: you can cultivate a habit of paying attention, a habit of catching your first response. Then you can build your directions into a coherent, balanced whole, whose momentum you can maintain with progressively smaller inputs of intent and attention than when you first learn the procedure. This takes time, more than you might think. All the attachments that hang off our 'saying no'—thoughts, attitudes, beliefs, emotional baggage—are up for the application of inhibition.

Traditional procedures can help us, both during training and after, to

- Build a back (meaning: strength arising out of good use);
- Strengthen oppositional pulls and our understanding of them;
- Cultivate our elasticity;
- Develop endurance in the application of inhibition and direction;

---

65 A Japanese martial arts teaching and training approach to embodying good technique in movement.

- Become more sensitive to the experience of expansion versus compression; and
- Reveal stuck places, where something restricts elasticity.

Most importantly, as teachers, traditional procedures can help us understand the process involved in any and all of the preceding points.

Working on yourself

At first, whether while using traditional procedures or more generally, all you might notice is when you are doing worse: increasing what you don't want, for example, squashing your neck, holding your breath, tightening your legs. Then you may get to *not* increasing this interference. As you make this change, your sensitivity to what you are dealing with improves. You become more sensitive to going wrong, for example, when you contract in some way (tightening the neck, collapsing, interfering with your breathing, losing your ground etc.). At this point you recognise that there is a difference between your usual way and this more considered way, and that it constitutes a qualitative difference to your being. This sensitivity feeds back into the loop, allowing deeper inhibition, further increasing your sensitivity to going wrong (because you recognise that you don't like what it feels like). Gradually, you may start to realise that going wrong may be a great deal subtler than stiffening some part of your body. For example, it may involve the quality of your attention: drifting/too diffuse or being too tightly focussed.

It takes time to effectively implement inhibition and direction, to develop an entire 'sphere' of expansion. This sphere must include not only some version of elastic length through your back, but also the ground, your limbs, three-dimensionality and the quality of your attention. It takes time to appreciate the internal and external relationships which these encompass. Using traditional procedures and their variations provides a framework for establishing the sphere.

Implications for teaching

You may give lessons to a singer who wants to make a better sound or improve their breathing, a golfer who wants a better swing or someone who wants to be able to do their desk-based job without pain. Teaching responses in all these scenarios may be inherent in what you have learnt through your own more abstract practice and understanding of traditional procedures. You might actually teach a traditional procedure, or simply be informed by an understanding that has come through your own practice of traditional procedures. The following examples provide an overview of some possibilities.

Working through whispered ahs may offer the singer an experience of freer primary control relationships. As the state of the singer's primary control relationships improves— through less pulling down and more elasticity generally— they will gain more responsiveness and freedom in their breathing. They will also enjoy more elasticity in their soft palate and freer suspension of their larynx. All this will have a positive effect on their sound. Through teaching the whispered ah, you can indirectly convey principles and the singer will learn that these corresponding benefits are possible.

In a similar way, yet without necessarily teaching a traditional procedure, your understanding of primary control relationships through your own working with semi-flexion or hands on the back of a chair may inform how you work with a golfer, to demonstrate the possibility of freer legs and arms, and how they relate to each other, head–torso freedom and ground contact. The golfer's swing will become more powerful and accurate as a result of their improving general use. Initiating the swing with freedom and a more coordinated torso as well as the concomitant improvements—*not* interfering with the breath or ground contact—minimises interferences with the unfolding of the swing, all the way out through the arms and legs.

With your understanding of traditional procedures and the light they shed on the primary control relationships and ensuing quality of use, you can help a desk-based worker improve their general conditions of use. Perhaps you start with the quality of their attention to the task they are doing. A less laser-focussed attitude can help reduce the end-gaining effort and strain of being at work, as well as facilitating balance on the chair and allowing a more supported use of their arms and hands. Inter alia, this approach might or might not involve actually using the traditional procedures, such as whispered ahs, hands on the back of a chair, semi-flexion or lunge.

I am not advocating necessarily formally teaching pupils traditional procedures. And I certainly do not suggest that this is all there is to helping a singer, golfer, desk worker or anyone else. Far from it. But the more you deeply understand your own use, the better. This is what grappling with traditional procedures can clarify. Ideally, you as the teacher understand the connections between the procedures and the various activities a pupil may want help with. Revisiting these procedures from time to time can be illuminating and revealing. Working on traditional procedures can deepen your appreciation of what you are working with yourself and what your pupils may struggle with. It can promote a deeper underpinning for the challenges of teaching.

Why time?

Remember that time is of the essence of the contract... It took me years to reach a point that can be reached in a few weeks with the aid of any experienced teacher.

F. MATTHIAS ALEXANDER[66]

Inhibition and direction *are* skills, and skills are learnable, if we have the interest and desire. Learning to reliably apply the Alexander Technique in our own lives is aspirational—we can always improve our application of inhibition and direction and our use. This implies consistent application over time.

Pain, a strong motivator, can be a wonderful reminder to come back to inhibition and direction. For example, if you always tighten your neck in response to a stimulus, your weight of experience will tell you that tightening your neck is a necessity, irrespective of the pain it might cause. Not tightening your neck may be completely inconceivable; it is outside of the range of your experience. Realising that the tightening might be connected to the pain, and that it is you who is tightening, takes time. Then, realising that you can reroute your response takes a little more time. Building facility with *not tightening* your neck takes more time again.

The longer we work with inhibition and direction in our daily lives, the more deeply we can go into the business of 'control of human reaction'.[67] We can apply this across the full range of our activities, including beyond the obviously 'physical', potentially pain-inducing elements. For example, you may start to more clearly see your emotional responses such as anger or joy, with a boss, a partner, children or work colleagues. You

---

66 Alexander, *Use of the Self*, ix.
67 Alexander, *Use of the Self*, 26, 28, 54.

might notice that these responses form predictable patterns, just like your responses to 'physical' situations. Your emotional responses may become clearer to you as you acquire the skills needed to maintain distance from them. Distance afforded through inhibition enables you to see the response; to see it as a choice and not identify with it. You then realise that you can handle progressively more complex and demanding situations without losing your cool, level head, balance or integration. This takes practice, and practice takes time.

Elements affecting the amount of time may include how much we attend to ourselves, our capacity for paying attention, our level of interest or curiosity about the process, how much else is going on in our lives and what other demands there are on us (for example, from relationships, jobs and lifestyle). How good we want to become at controlling our reactions is another element. For example, you may be delighted with being able to control pain—the most common starting point for learning the Alexander Technique—and making it go away when it comes. For many, this is not such a high order of skill, often learnable in just a few weeks. But if you want to eliminate pain completely, this typically takes longer—maybe months or more. Improving your use is an open-ended process. Steering your use such that eventually use not only determines function, but that the cumulative imperceptible moment-to-moment 'resets' also affect structure, probably comes through years of paying attention. And this, of course, creates a progressively wider margin before pain becomes an issue.

When I started having Alexander Technique lessons, I had a marked lordosis and suffered lower back pain. Early lessons brought an immediate reduction in the frequency of pain. After about one year, I was pain-free much of the time, but some activities or emotional situations could still trigger the old patterns. As I continued to pay attention to my use, I started to see that under my physical-tension reactions lay emotional reactions to which inhibition could also be applied. Steadily, my back improved, pain gradually ceased to be an issue at all and the lordosis quietly disappeared. Working with this process and rerouting my habitual maladaptive responses took time.

Teaching-related time

Many people play a musical instrument at an amateur level. There are many extremely good amateur players. What's the difference between the amateur and the professional musician? One is a consistency and predictability in the professional's minimum level of competence. That is, the worst that they would play on a bad day is still acceptable, and good enough to be paid for. Attaining a professional level of competence generally takes years and is achieved through formal practice, of scales, technical drills, studies and pieces. It takes consistent intent to work on all the necessary elements, lots of listening to themselves during practice, and exposure to a variety of music in a wide range of circumstances. There are no shortcuts to the time it takes.

Similarly, to become a beginning-level teacher of the Alexander Technique, and to then develop depth as a teacher, requires a deal of attention to your own use of your self. This includes attention to all the material that you learn when you first start having lessons:

· Cultivating an applied, practical understanding of the basic ideas, traditionally expressed as use, the primary control, inhibition and direction;

· Learning some practical anatomy, including understanding how it relates to your own use of your self, and clearing up any body-mapping misconceptions;

- Paying attention to how you use your self in your daily life; this may start to extend beyond the physical; and
- Applying inhibition and direction in attitude, relationships, decision-making and other situations.

All this takes a while. And the aspiring Alexander Technique teacher needs to cover all of this and take it further. As an Alexander teacher, you need to

- Understand how all of the foregoing relates to communicating inhibition and direction, both verbally and with your hands;
- Learn to listen with your hands as well as perceive with your ears and eyes;
- Understand how to work on yourself and cultivate a long-term attitude to that, regarding any and every situation as an opportunity to work on yourself;
- Match what you say and do, to the pupil you are addressing in a lesson;
- Say enough yet not too much;
- Leave distractions outside your teaching room; and
- Put all of this together coherently.[68]

These are high-order skills. It takes time to become consistent, reliable and adequately competent at a beginning-teacher level. After training, if we keep paying attention and practising what we preach, we can spend the rest of our lives improving, refining and honing what we do and how we do it.

There is a story about a mathematics professor who is explaining something complex which he writes on the blackboard for his students. He points to a part of the workings and says, 'This is obvious.' Then he pauses anxiously, suddenly

---

68 See 'The teaching journey—A lifelong exploration', page 106.

wondering if it is, in fact, obvious. He goes to his office and covers many sheets of paper in close calculations before returning some time later, looking relieved and saying, 'Yes, it is obvious.' As we progress with the work, our understanding deepens. It can be very useful to check our assumptions and what we think is obvious. Do others share our assumptions? 'Is this still what I think it is?'

For Alexander Technique teachers who focus just on freeing the neck, maybe the whole thing is obvious and self-evident. Maybe they can, like FM himself, convey something whether their pupil is interested or not. However, most of us benefit from a broader understanding and from being able to build a coherent, internally logical picture in which the primary control interrelationships[69] are clear. Perhaps it's all only obvious once we have done the work, and this takes time.

---

69 Consider not only the extent of the primary control interrelationships — for example, between 'head forward and up' and 'knees forward and away', which entirely depend on 'back lengthening and widening/back to stay back' and so on — but also the circularity of the non-doing quality of inhibition and direction, and how each element plays into and is reflected by all the others.

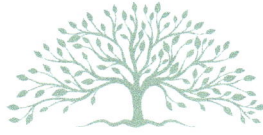

CHAPTER 4

General specifics and practical explorations

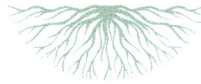

[We practise FM's traditional procedures not to be] backward-looking but to deepen our understanding of the fundamental principles and practices underlying the technique and improve the application of these in our own times. Without these insights another danger to the ongoing transmission of the technique is that Alexander practitioners won't know why they are doing what they are doing. In which case it will be inevitable that some teachers will question many aspects of the Alexander enterprise, perhaps concluding that activities, such as chair and table work, going on to the toes or the whispered ah are pointless, historically situated rituals which ought to be replaced with practices more in tune with a post-modern zeitgeist. But that, I submit, would be like throwing out the baby (and the bath) with the bathwater.

SEÁN CAREY[70]

---

70 Carey, *Think More, Do Less*, 13.

At the beginning of 1986, when I had been qualified less than a year, I attended my first workshop with Marj Barstow. Hers was a very different way of working from how I had been trained. I tried to relate her way of working to what I then understood. After one morning session, having not yet heard her mention a word signifying what I had understood to be a key element in the Alexander Technique, I asked, 'Marj, what about inhibition?' With a smile, she replied, 'Whaddaya think we've been working on?' Without being named, inhibition had been implicit. To get to implicit, however, we need to start with explicit.

In this chapter, I describe some of Alexander's traditional procedures and what the practice of each may bring. I include other 'games' as well. Generally, they represent great vehicles for self-work—practising inhibition and direction with the goal of more activated primary control relationships. This chapter may be most relevant to trainees and new teachers. However, established teachers may find useful morsels here too. I also offer brief ideas for practical explorations while working with procedures. Play with these on your own (you can record and play back the instructions) or with a colleague, who can read the instructions and/or assist you with hands-on guidance.[71] Remember that in all this, inhibition needs to be explicit before it can become implicit.

But first, a few words about ground contact, which plays into all the practical explorations that follow.

Ground

There is a poetic martial arts idea about posture which says that the head should be suspended 'between heaven and earth'.

---

71   See also 'Why traditional procedures?', page 44.

After an Alexander lesson, pupils sometimes mention feeling grounded, that their legs feel light or that they are floating as they walk. These apparently contradictory comments are about the experience of how we process our weight. This is what we are doing all the time—processing and dealing with our weight. That is, we are managing our response to gravity, whether we are moving or still.

A super-bouncy ball is a fair metaphor for the way we use weight and contact. The ball changes direction when it hits a hard surface; it bounces much less on a soft surface. Walking any distance on dry sand or in deep snow, where we have nothing firm to respond to, is effortful. Similarly, it is more difficult to be 'up' in a soft armchair than on a hard kitchen stool. It is our contact with the planet or a proxy (like a chair) that informs our processes of 'uprighting' (our built-in organisation of postural management). Gravity is a given. Paying attention to the resulting contact that we have with our supporting surfaces is basic to optimising our use. 'Head forward and up, back lengthening and widening, and knees forward and away' all bear a relation to the ground and our contact with it. Thus, contact has to be a constant theme. 'Up' is relative to the ground.

Grounded doesn't mean down

'Grounded' is sometimes interpreted to mean a downward energy, a felt heaviness. This needs careful qualification. Grounded certainly refers to the ground beneath, something which is down or below us. What goes down, however, is only weight, through the essentially weight-bearing parts: our bones, along with any associated soft tissue. The weight must travel through the bones freely, unhindered by unnecessary muscular holding. This absolutely includes the legs.

To the extent that we can balance ourselves through our bones, including those of the lower limbs, and not brace or hold ourselves up muscularly, our muscles are available for the delicate maintenance and adjustment of this balance. This is also true through constant movement, including breathing, walking, running, or fine movements like those involved in playing a musical instrument. Consider the qualitative contrast between the average, young, strong, gym junkie versus a top dancer, horse rider or rock climber—the latter group can summon light, coordinated strength without excessive muscular holding. Considering this minimum of muscular activity, enough to keep the whole balanced and responsive but not more, as needed by any top performer, is another way of thinking about the quality of elastic responsiveness discussed elsewhere.[72] If we attempt to achieve 'up' without attention to the ground, we become tight and stiff, with restricted breathing.

Gravity is our friend. Postural support is related to how we respond to gravity. It can be interesting to ponder the considerable effort it takes astronauts to adopt a 'straight' posture, for example, standing or sitting erect, in the absence of gravity. Without gravity bringing us into contact with a firm surface, we are bereft of relevant information our nervous system needs in order to organise posture. Astronauts lose bone density and suffer other health problems in the absence of gravity. Roger Tengwall concluded that we need gravity to trigger fully upright posture.[73]

---

72 See 'Primary control relationships', page 11; and the details on legs under 'Semi-flexion', page 59.
73 See Roger Warren Tengwall, "On Human Postural Behaviours" (PhD diss., University of California, Irvine, 1981).

Semi-flexion

Semi-flexion[74] is an Alexander Technique procedure used to work on one's use. Well performed, semi-flexion results in an overall balance of gravity-related, toned elasticity which may be clearer than in any other attitude. It comprises a concise, practical 'digest' of the primary control relationships. This study of relationships then informs any other position, movement or reaction. Semi-flexion puts a demand on your ability to maintain the necessary directions as a conscious act. Effective semi-flexion depends on your ability to keep applying multiple strands of inhibition and direction, an attentional juggling act that cultivates an expanded field of attention to Alexander's various oppositional pulls—for example, back lengthening versus legs releasing out—to produce a light, elastic, responsive state of being. Semi-flexion can clarify how the oppositional pulls reinforce one another, bringing you towards a state and quality of dynamic balance which can be endlessly refined.

Semi-flexion is commonly misunderstood as a generic term for any *position* that is upright with hips, knees and ankles partially flexed. However, this misses the point: the quality of postural *tone* is paramount. The point is to cultivate responsive, dynamic, toned, elastic expansion throughout, whatever the position or degree of flexion.[75]

What's it good for?

Working on the cultivation of reliable, coordinated, elastic semi-flexion starts and continues the development of

- A good working position for teaching;

---

74 This was formerly referred to as 'monkey'.
75 See Carey, *Think More, Do Less*, 113.

- A 'good' integrated back, including pelvis, spine, rib cage and scapulae, and associated musculature;
- A constructive relationship between the head, torso, all four limbs and the ground;
- Breathing that is integrated into the primary control; and
- The vital and consequential capacity to sustain inhibition and expanding, elastic oppositional direction.

Wrapping your head around semi-flexion also asks for clarity—deep thinking about how you are using your self and why, getting you to grapple with your internal and external relationships. This latter may involve examining the quality of your attention—is it narrower than it could be? Is it more vague (relaxed) than is useful?[76] Where is the sweet spot for the quality of your attention, bearing in mind that you are moving it all the time? With your attention, can you encompass yourself, what you are engaged in, plus your environment, for example, the person you are working with, the room you are in, the view?

Semi-flexion and why we use the chair in teaching

Consider semi-flexion in relation to the use of the chair in teaching. John Nicholls points out that one reason we use a chair, as FM did, is that it replicates a truncated version of the movement we stereotypically make as young toddlers; standing up, then squatting, followed by coming up again, all in service of being able to explore our environment.[77] At that early age, we establish and exercise a set of working relationships. This includes balancing a heavy head with coordinating support through the trunk, then balancing head and trunk

---

76 Irene Tasker uses the word 'drift' in her notes: 'The other extreme of too hasty reaction is drift.' Stratil, *Irene Tasker*, 258.

77 John Nicholls and Seán Carey, *The Alexander Technique: In Conversation with John Nicholls and Seán Carey* (Redwood Press Limited, 1991), 66-68

over the legs, which fold and unfold to get us down or up, and articulate to move us around. Using the chair in teaching effectively revisits this territory of the working relationships between head, torso and legs. Apart from replicating a developmental stage, using the chair in a lesson provides a template which can be applied generally. It incorporates attentiveness, inhibition, direction and using accurate concepts mapped onto actual physiology.

Is it actually semi-flexion?

Believing that one is wonderfully semi-flexing, while in reality not doing so, is the easiest thing in the world. Rather than simply adopting a position, semi-flexion is about directing the underlying relationships such that they foster lively expansion throughout the framework. Many years ago, a former long-time pupil, who was then training elsewhere to become an Alexander teacher, demonstrated to me guiding a fellow trainee into semi-flexion. He pointed out what good semi-flexion she was achieving. His fellow trainee happened to be someone whose joints articulated fairly freely. Her use was not apparently terrible; she was in a reasonable state. Her semi-flexion looked alright from the outside, but when I put my hands on her, I found that it was actually devoid of any lively energy on the inside. It had no elasticity or bounce, no reference to the floor and little 'up'. She was semi-flexing very much out of her stiff, habitual use, with no real lift in her energetic direction and, therefore, no expansion. Her thinking was not engaged in an adequately inhibitory way, nor was there much quality of aspiration for elastic lengthening in her direction. So while it superficially looked like semi-flexion, the whole thing was 'dead', energy-less. As both trainees were just part-way through their training, neither had yet realised that something essential was missing. A triumph of form over content, it missed the point entirely.

We always need to assume that there are elements in our own use (and that of our pupils) that we simply do not see or recognise. Misuse may, at times, create downstream limits or deficiencies in our function, yet we remain blind to their origins. For example, it is easy to get into a habit in semi-flexion that involves subtly tightening down into the hip joints. This would be associated with slight undue tension in the legs, with the torso limited to being only partially energised and awake. This less than optimal pattern would simultaneously restrict freedom of the breath. Attention that awakens the legs, such that they have a dynamic relationship to the floor and the torso—i.e., preventing habitual stiffening—seems to be an aspect of use that even some qualified teachers have not discovered, nor worked through. In fact, I had not either, until it was explicitly explained and shown to me, a couple of years into my teaching career. What a difference it made everywhere! My arms and hands became so much freer and more responsive.

This relationship between torso and legs has implications: for the breath, and for the support and aliveness of the arms and hands as well as of the legs. Not taking this relationship into account results in a reduced quality of contact with the ground. This contact also feeds directly back into the quality of your direction. Heavy, tree-trunk legs do not spring off the ground and do not assist in mobile liveliness for the hands, breath or anything else. When everything is working well, it is as though the ground comes up through your feet and legs and informs your whole torso, head and arms with direction. This ground-informed upward direction may also be experienced as a 'keying in' of the abdominal contents towards the spine, as the floating ribs are activated. Greater freedom in your legs and effective ground contact may make it feel as though your internal organs stay better connected towards your back, opposing your legs and arms, which can release out. This may also be expressed as a dynamic opposition of the diaphragm and legs releasing away from one another as the floating ribs are activated. Free and proper movement of the diaphragm is facilitated when, subjectively, the viscera are not being pulled forward and down/the legs are not being pulled in[78] — rather, the back of the pelvis is allowed to widen. This freer diaphragmatic movement may also be experienced as a slight toning from the pubic symphysis towards the sternum, or the merest hint of a 'pointing' of the coccyx forward. A further concomitant is a freeing of the ribs, which may also be experienced as described earlier. The key point remains: the relationship between torso and legs is reciprocal. Any tightening in the torso, meaning restricting of the breath, instantly degrades the freedom in the legs, and vice versa.[79,80]

---

78 I use the slash here to indicate that these two elements are different descriptions of the same pattern.

79 This paragraph is an attempt to describe experiences. They probably have much to do with an evenness of tone throughout the abdominal wall, including the pelvic floor and the dorsal parts. Note that this may be the antithesis of 'engaging the core' or doing abdominal exercises. See Barlow and Davies, *Examined Life*, 64:

> FM used to say that 'neck free, head forward and up, back to lengthen and widen' was the nearest he could get in words to what couldn't be put into words. He used to say, 'It's rotten really, it's no good, but it's the best...I can do.... It's the nearest I can get in words to the experience you need to have.'

80 See Alexander, *Man's Supreme Inheritance*, 115:

> During the practical process by which the thoracic elasticity and maximum intra-thoracic capacity are gradually established, the body of the subject is at the same time readjusted, and mental principles are inculcated which will enable him to maintain the improved conditions in posture and co-ordination which are being set up, and which will secure the normal and necessary abdominal pressure in the right direction, thus constituting a natural form of massage of the digestive organs which is maintained during the ordinary actions of everyday life.

Universal constants

Whatever attitude or position we are in, our primary control relationships remain. As long as you have a head, neck, back and limbs, there are relationships between them. They are a constant, for good or for ill. The ground contact—with the back (semi-supine), hands and knees (all fours) or feet (upright standing or semi-flexion)—is also a constant that informs these key relationships. The different positions may throw new light on the meanings of the relationships, allowing us to verbalise how we want them to be.[81] For example, 'neck free, head forward and out'[82] when on all fours demands a well-toned back, a condition which also corresponds to breathing that involves properly distributed muscular tone. This can thus illuminate the meaning of 'neck free, head forward and out' when in any other attitude, such as standing, semi-flexion or walking.

A danger in semi-supine is that we can slip into passivity. When lying down we need to remain alive, toned and attentive. Direction and intent need to be based in active attention. The same is true in any position (think of any position as being transitional, i.e., on the way to somewhere else). All fours also requires active tone throughout, as the whole torso responds to floor contact. This same contact-activated, primary control-steered tone applies equally in standing, walking, going onto the toes or anything else. Each position can inform all of the others—the primary control relationships remain constant.

---

81 Directions are an attempt to describe in words the relationships that we want.

82 'Forward and out' as opposed to 'forward and up' seems much more logical to me when in semi-supine, or on all fours. In any degree of flexion, 'forward and out' also seems more accurate and easier to understand than 'forward and up'.

Practical explorations: Semi-flexion via semi-supine, all fours and standing

In this section, I offer a way of working, in a practical sequence that moves from semi-supine, via all fours and standing, to semi-flexion (Explorations 1–8). All the way through, the sequence attends to the key relationships which define the primary control. As we work through different positions, the relationships between parts persist. Take your time trying out the following suggestions. As you work your way through, remember that awake non-reactivity, i.e., inhibition, is your friend.

You may wish to record yourself reading the instructions for each exploration.[83]

---

83 Alternatively, audio guides for the explorations are being gradually added at https://freedominaction.com.au/resources/.

A note on the figures

The illustrations on the next pages are not definitive. They are presented, rather, as two-dimensional models, with each one open to amendment and development. The models should not be confused with reality. Indeed, two apparently inconsistent images might both be true. Note that the quickest and most direct way to check intended meanings is probably through practical, hands-on work.

The nature of directions, represented by arrows in the illustrations, is that they describe relationships. The relationships hold good all the time. If you want good, oppositionally elastic use, then you need to satisfy 'neck free, head forward and up' and so on, whether you sit, move to standing, stand, move to sitting, crawl on all fours, sit at your desk, run up a hill or anything else. Similarly, for fully oppositionally elastic use, 'knees forward and away' must be satisfied, whatever you are doing. Ideally, there is no discontinuity in the aliveness[84] of the relationships/directions at any point. Note that if we flip the semi-flexed figure by 90 degrees, to semi-supine, all the arrows remain valid and applicable. If we then flip it 180 degrees to all fours, again, the arrows are still valid.

The directions describe something that is inherent to the nature of the parts and their relationships to their neighbours. They could be considered interrelated concomitants. For example, 'knees forward and away' implies certain other things.[85] When standing upright, it means the need for opposition between legs and torso: legs releasing out of the trunk implies

---

84 'Aliveness' relates to attention and its quality. It bespeaks a receptive, non-reactive quality of attentiveness. It is constantly coming and going, and is thus aspirational.
85 See 'Is it actually semi-flexion?', page 61.

freedom in the joints and freedom to move, if you don't tighten as you begin to move. Not restricting the movement of the ribs is a concomitant. When straightening up, for example, out of a chair or from a bend, the knees still need to retain the forward and away relationship to the torso, notwithstanding that the knees are actually moving backwards in space. That is, we don't want to unduly contract the legs—neither pulling the knees back nor losing the ground connection by tightening the calves or feet. Instead, we want a movement in which the leg muscles continue to lengthen as the legs straighten. In this sort of movement, for example, coming up out of a squat or out of semi-flexion, attention to releasing the heels away from the bottom/sitting bones is also an expression of 'knees forward and away' and can be helpful. If this direction—inadequately summarised in the phrase 'knees forward and away'—is achieved, then an associated, continuing freedom in the lower back, including the floating ribs, is simultaneously available, as is continuing freedom in the breath and the legs.

Arrow key

For visual clarity, I generally do not include arrows indicating basic directions, whatever form they take for you. Rather, I address their essential concomitants, which explicate the basic directions.

Red: The red lines denote ground contact. The red arrowheads denote what can be triggered via the ground contact—applying quiet intention and preparedness for the head forward and out, recognising that this relates to an intention for length along the entire spine. This means giving your weight freely down to the ground contact and coming up off it. There is an overall opposition between the red lines and the red arrowheads. This applies equally in semi-supine, all fours and when you are on your feet.

Green: Include the legs—they contribute liveliness to the primary control relationships. These arrows represent more or less 'particular' directions—things to include in your attention. The arrow pointing around the buttocks does *not* signify a tuck. The arrow across the back of the belt line indicates length and breadth throughout the lower back, i.e., breathing, including freedom of the floating ribs and volume of the entire pelvis. This allows release around the buttocks and length along the backs of the thighs. It indicates an unclenching release which includes allowing the whole pelvis to undo away (up) from the femoral heads or vice versa. This simultaneously feeds the forward knee direction and is analogous to length along the calves—between the backs of the knees and the heels and floor. That is, release both in thighs and in calves can feed the forward knee direction.

Purple (all fours and rocking): The purple arrows represent length along the torso, with full excursion of the ribs, recognising the associated gentle displacement of all abdominal organs. It includes allowing this displacement into the entire volume of the pelvis, right down to the pelvic floor, without losing the integrity/tone of the torso as a whole (see Figure 2).

Purple (standing and semi-flexion): These arrows indicate a general opposition between torso and legs. Maintain length along the torso, as before. This may clarify something of how the torso and legs stay away from each other, which can be expressed as 'knees forward and away' (see the green arrows—not losing the integrity of the torso as a whole; see Figure 4).

Light blue (all fours and rocking): The light blue arrows denote whole torso up off the ground contacts.

Blue: Referring to overall length and springiness, the blue arrow encompasses everything and, therefore, includes the ideas depicted by the other colours.

The layers of colour are an attempt to represent both a closer view (the shorter arrows) and the overall view (the longer arrows). It is worth remembering that in working on ourselves, we need to take in both views simultaneously. We could always add further layers, both close-up and wide-angle views.

Exploration 1: Semi-supine — Floor contact informs the intent for length/breadth/volume

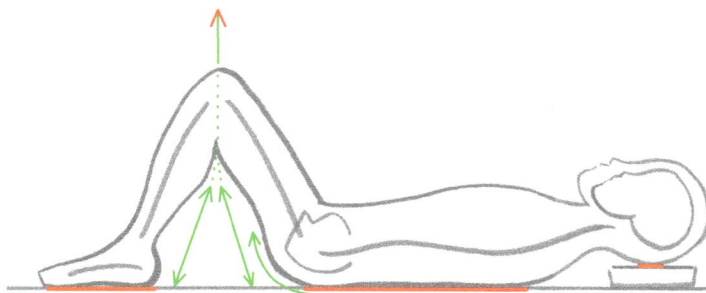

Figure 1. Semi-supine

Note the intention for the knees towards the ceiling, which is the resultant of heels/knees and pelvis/knees, as per the green arrows.

Lie in semi-supine:

- Becoming quiet, open to what is, including contact with your supporting surface;
- Exercising an attitude of open, non-judgemental receptivity; and
- Including your breath in your attention.

Now bring forward the background of intent of your directions:

- Neck free, head forward and out, back to lengthen and widen;
- This means having your eyes open and alive to what you see, for example, the ceiling and what's around you;
- Orient towards length and three-dimensional volume throughout your torso. Along with the ongoing intent for a free neck to allow the head its forward and outward direction relative to a lengthening and widening back, this means the intent to allow gentle displacement of your viscera towards the base of your pelvis with each in-breath, including around your full circumference. There is no great demand for air when in semi-supine, but you want the freedom available so that your breathing can be responsive to potential demand;

- Orient your knees towards the ceiling,[86] which means a preparedness for
  - Allowing a softer breadth across the back of your pelvis/freedom of movement of the floating ribs[87] and the ribs in general;
  - The muscular wrapping of the thigh bones to soften;
  - Asking for length from the back of your pelvis, including the sitting bones, around your bottom and up the back of your thighs (not a tuck; see the green arrows);
  - Allowing length through the backs of the lower legs, from heels to backs of the knees. Inhabiting the lower legs with your thinking in this way can help to gradually enliven your legs; and
  - Breathing, which may feel like an opposition between your diaphragm/back of your ribs and your legs. The more freely you breath, the freer your legs become, and vice versa.

Remember that in semi-supine we want an awake, toned state, no less than when we are upright and active. Including the legs, as described earlier, feeds into the other directions and can help to make them more responsive too. Through all this, don't become attached to feeling anything in particular!

Before moving from semi-supine to all fours, first 'see' yourself in the new position in your mind's eye, as per the following paragraph. Only then, roll over onto all fours.

---

86 See Carey, *Think More, Do Less*, 148.
87 Here, while including the entire rib cage, I highlight the floating ribs. This is because while there may be movement of the ribs in general, full activation of the floating ribs is often missed. When the floating ribs are available for movement, there is less downward pressure of the torso towards the legs and greater freedom for the viscera to be gently displaced downwards, as needed, as the ribs swing out and the diaphragm descends. The legs may also become freer.

Exploration 2: All fours — Opposition between torso, including pelvis, and limbs

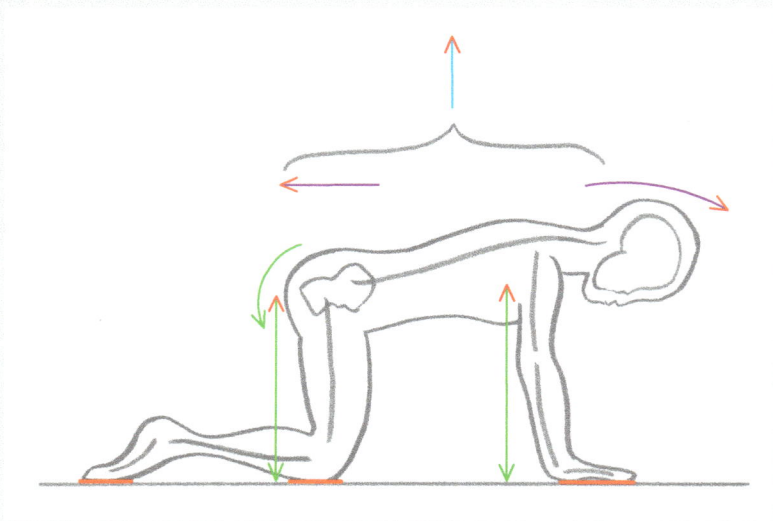

Figure 2. All fours[88]

All fours is roughly an upside-down version of semi-supine, with the addition of support through the arms. Note the same principle as in semi-supine: you can respond to the contacts with the planet by expanding off them. Whereas in semi-supine you want the knees pointing at the ceiling, in opposition to the back, on all fours, the whole back/torso is directed back and up off the legs and the arms, in opposition to the hand and knee contact. You can still use 'neck free, back lengthening and widening' etc. as your directions — they remain true. And it may be clearer to think in the following terms: opposition between the whole three-dimensional torso and the ground contacts through your hands, knees and dorsal feet. This means the whole torso springs up off the ground contacts, all of which facilitates the breath, which feeds the 'up' off the ground contacts and promotes length. Being on all fours, with good use, more clearly asks for the toned state of quiet readiness that you cultivated in semi-supine. And the relationships framed in your directions remain identical. Note the notional opposition between the breath-activated back of ribs and

88   All fours may not be a traditional procedure, but it can provide a valuable transition between semi-supine and being on your feet.

waist versus the knees out of the torso. That is, both positions, semi-supine and all fours, maintain a lively opposition between torso and legs (see Figures 1 and 2).

When on all fours, the knees need to have about a spread hand's breadth of space between them (i.e., knees below hip joints) and the toes should be extended. With both rocking and crawling, a key point is to use the floor contact to expand up off, with the whole torso toning, rather than collapsing between the arms and legs, fixing, or collapsing between the scapulae. It should not feel like your hands are carrying an undue weight. Your wrists may be directly under your shoulders. But if your wrists object to this, place your hands further forward. Note that width across your back provides support. This includes width between the scapulae, with the ribs, including the floating ribs, supporting the scapulae, while still allowing free rib movement for the breath. Your whole torso can continue to spring, via your arms and legs, off the contacts that you have with the floor, principally your hands and knees. You can also include the contacts of your shins and dorsal feet in your attention. Your head is still prepared to lead (see the purple arrows), your back can continue to lengthen and widen, and your three-dimensional torso continues to be breathed, from the base of your skull to the base of your pelvis. Note that it is usually easier to work through all of this while moving gently in a backward and forward rocking motion.[89]

---

89 These instructions are more or less generic. Allowance may need to be made, and closer attention given, for any particular individual, for example, if you are kyphotic or hypermobile.

Exploration 3: Rocking — Torso/limb opposition, releasing the legs more and allowing the ribs to move

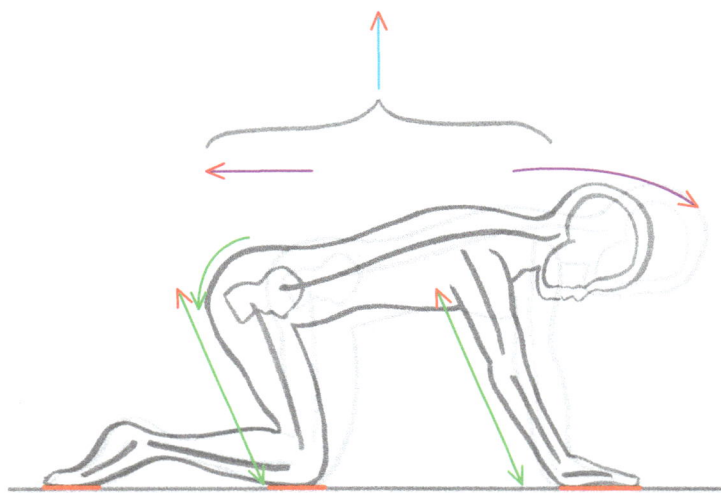

Figure 3. Rocking on all fours

Gently start to rock by moving *backwards* from your neutral start position, then rock forwards again. Come forward only as far as your start position, i.e., with no acute angle at the wrists, to minimise discomfort in those joints. Elbows remain unlocked. (Hypermobile individuals: take note of both these points.) Aim for a gentle, rhythmical, smooth rocking movement, initiated and maintained via your direction, rather than by 'muscling'. A typical backward–forward cycle might take about two seconds.

Once you get comfortable with this, consider the muscles running from the back of your sitting bones, around your bottom, to the backs of your knees. Ask for release in these muscles, both while going backwards and going forwards, enlivening your intention for release between your pelvis and legs. Work with this direction, perhaps daily for several days or a week, without ignoring other elements of your primary control relationships. Then consider asking for release in the lower legs — from the backs of the knees through the calves, across the fronts of the ankles and out to your toes — on every *forward* part of the cycle. All the while, of course, maintaining your usual directions, however you frame them. For example, neck free, head forward and out, back to lengthen and widen, and torso up off the arms and legs. Keep an eye on your breathing, continuing to activate your back 'back'. Again, the relationships all remain — nothing changes.

Working with the preceding directions (releasing around your bottom and backs of thighs to knees, and releasing calves while going forwards), in this relatively unfamiliar attitude of rocking on all fours, may be comparatively less hindered by a depth of habit associated with semi-supine, standing or walking. Thus, this may provide a route to realising clearer fundamental primary control relationships in standing and semi-flexion.

To come up to your feet from all fours, curl your toes under and walk your hands back towards your knees. Then roll back and up onto your feet, coming up to your full height, paying attention to the available oppositional length between your head and heels, i.e., don't pull your head back or down, or tighten your legs. Release your heels down as you come up.

Exploration 4: Standing upright

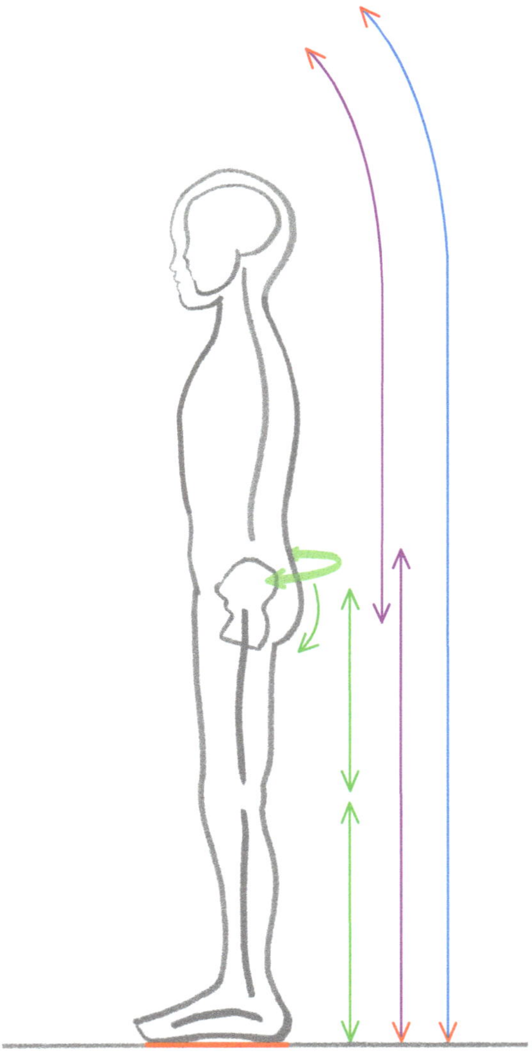

Figure 4. Standing upright

Once you are standing fully upright, all of your directions can continue, particularly with respect to your legs. This again means an intention for opposition between your head and ground contact, and continuing to work with the other relationships. Note (and see the purple arrows)

- The opposition between your legs and torso/breathing: your torso[90] back and up relative to your legs; floating ribs active; legs away out of your lower back/groin/front crease of hip joints; and the viscera off the legs, all while standing erect; and
- The length from the back of your pelvis, around your bottom, through the backs of your thighs in particular, to the backs of your knees, and then from the backs of your knees to heels (see the green arrows).

Do not compress/contract

- Your neck;
- The length and volume of your torso;
- The backs of your thighs;
- Your calves; or
- Your widening back (note your breathing).

As your floating ribs become freer, your abdomen tones and presses down less. Any and all of this contributes to conditions for the breathing to become freer — for it to 'do itself'. Notwithstanding your change in position to upright, the relationships remain the same. It may feel different. Yet all that has changed is your position — the working relationships, as before, still need to continue.

---

90 When teaching, I may use the words 'back', 'torso', 'body' and 'trunk' interchangeably, depending on the context. A key function of the entire back/torso/body/trunk is to encompass the process of moving air in and out. Thus, there is an intimate overlap between the back/torso/body/trunk and the function of breathing.

Semi-flexion

When you contemplate going from standing upright to semi-flexion, none of the preceding directions/relationships needs to change. In fact, find a way of moving to semi-flexion such that you lose none of the clarity of the relationships: between head and torso; and torso, legs and breath. Your knees can freely ease forwards (with no constraint on the freedom of your breath) as your upper body effortlessly tips forward and hip joints move back. The balance doesn't change over your feet, and your breathing continues unrestricted, as before.

- The act of moving to semi-flexion may need to include plenty of inhibition of the habitual. You may need to give a lot of attention to continuing to release around your bottom and the backs of your legs to the floor, as well as to not constraining your breathing, nor shortening up and down the front of the hip joints or lower abdomen. It may feel unfamiliar.

When you are in semi-flexion, all of these directions continue, particularly with respect to the legs.

- Along with an overall 'up', continue with the intent for length through the backs of your thighs, and between the knees and the heels (feet open to the floor), while maintaining your background directions for your neck/head/torso/breath.

Something to ponder

The semi-flexion arrows in Figures 5–7 would be familiar to many. However, what do they mean in the process of uprighting from semi-flexion, and in the process of being fully erect? Recognise that it is a process. When we are fully erect—and 'going up'—how do our directions relate to any position other than fully erect? While there is not much movement, there are still micro-adjustments, unlike for an object on a shelf. How do the directions apply? What is their quality?

Exploration 5: Slight semi-flexion

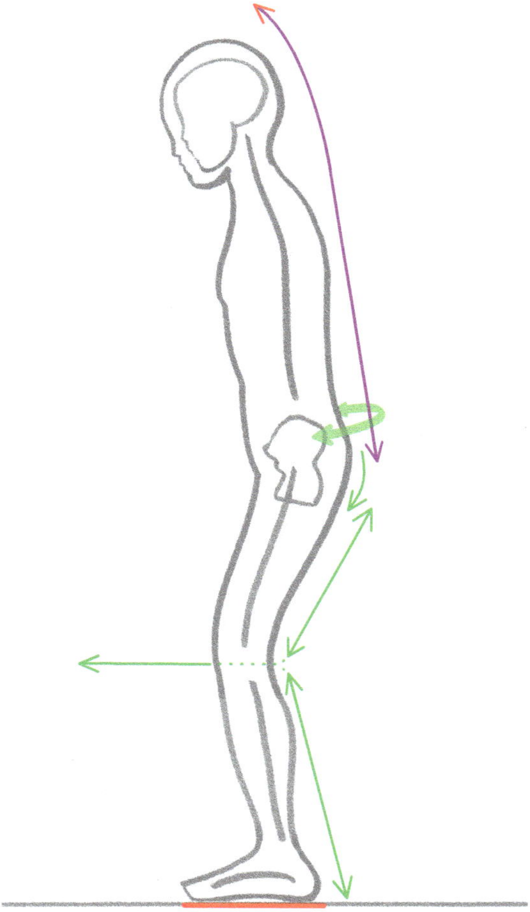

Figure 5. Slight semi-flexion

All directions related to Figure 4 continue to apply. Optimising your use is still driven by opposition between your head direction and floor contact, and all of the concomitants. For example, neck free, head forward and out, back to lengthen and widen, not tightening the legs and breath working freely. This means that you attend to and work with whatever restrictions are relevant to you at the time.

- Keep opening your feet to the floor while maintaining a gentle intent for your head forward and out;
- Continue allowing length around your bottom towards the backs of your thighs;
- Release the backs of your legs into length; and
- Don't forget to breathe.

You are three-dimensional. Acknowledge not only the length at the back, front and sides of your thorax, but also observe and allow the gentle displacement of all your abdominal organs downwards, including towards the pelvic floor. Consider the three-dimensional volume of your abdomen, including availability of the entire volume of your pelvis. Also, there is the volume afforded by the free movement of the floating ribs, which has the effect of supporting the abdominal contents back and up towards your spine. When you move from standing erect, with minimal effort, to semi-flexion, nothing needs to change in these relationships and the consequent quality of expansion.

Exploration 6: Slightly deeper semi–flexion

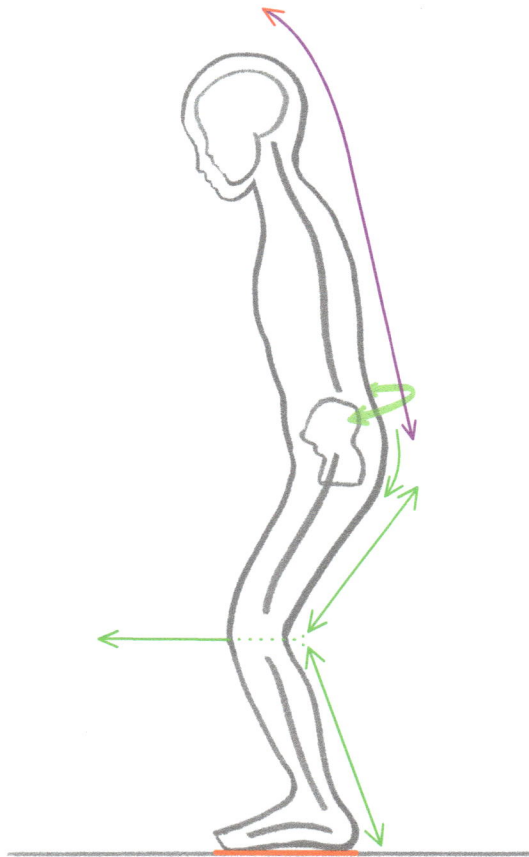

Figure 6. Slightly deeper semi–flexion

As before, continue to consider your floor contact versus your head and note your breath.

Again, all comments from the previous explorations continue to apply. Pay attention to giving weight through free legs and open feet to the floor, simultaneously with allowing the floor up through the channels of your legs. That is, continue to not grip your legs, particularly the backs of them. You are still not pulling your head in or down, and do allow the breath to continue freely, i.e., not denying any of the potential 'displacement volume' for your internal organs, gently to the floor of your pelvis.[91]

---

91   See the description in Exploration 5: Slight semi-flexion, page 81.

Exploration 7: Deep semi-flexion

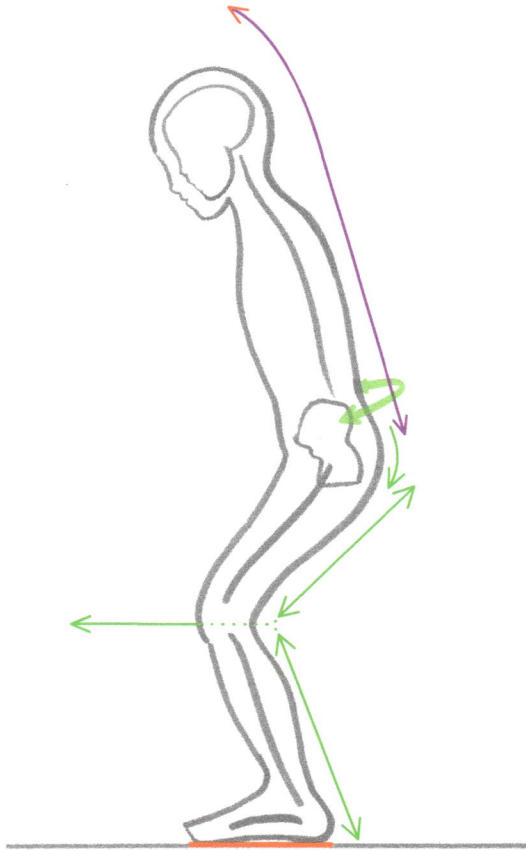

Figure 7. Deep semi-flexion

Like all directions, the knee direction does not exist by itself. It comes about as a consequence of releasing the backs of the legs, such that the knees can move freely forwards, in the continuing context of all the other directions.[92]

The context of the other directions brings us straight back to 'head forward and out', which can't truly happen without 'neck free', which relates to allowing the entire torso its proper length, breadth and depth. This depends on not tightening the legs, allowing an open contact with the floor, which informs the neck and head. And around we go yet again!

---

92 The fronts of the thighs tend more or less to take care of themselves if we attend to the backs of the thighs.

Exploration 8: Semi-flexion to fully upright

Still nothing changes in the primary control relationships. In the act of returning to orthograde standing from semi-flexion, still *continue to continue* with the same directions. Don't tighten your legs or around your buttocks. Your legs continue to lengthen/release, the ground contact and breathing can remain completely undisturbed, as can the freedom along the full length of your spine, including your neck.

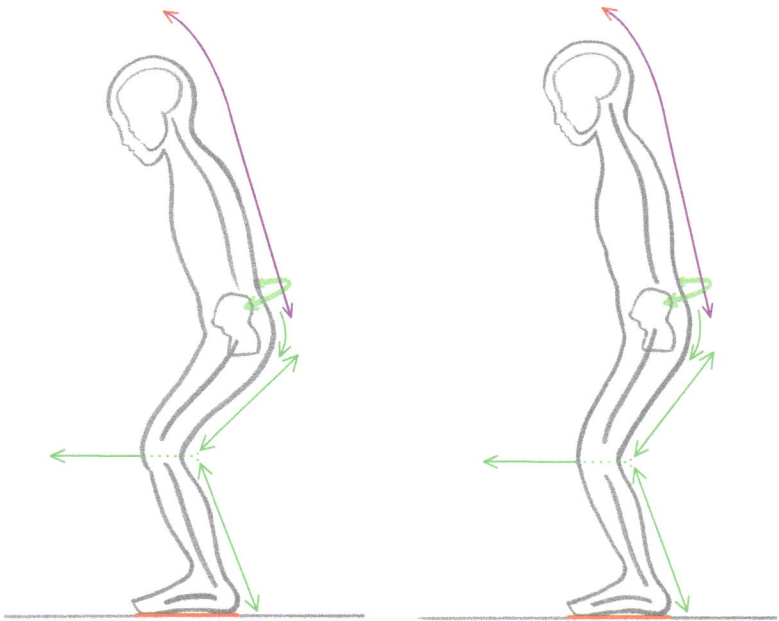

Figure 8. Semi-flexion to standing

We aspire to attend to all these directions/relationships, whatever position we are in, whatever movement we make and whatever our surrounding circumstances.

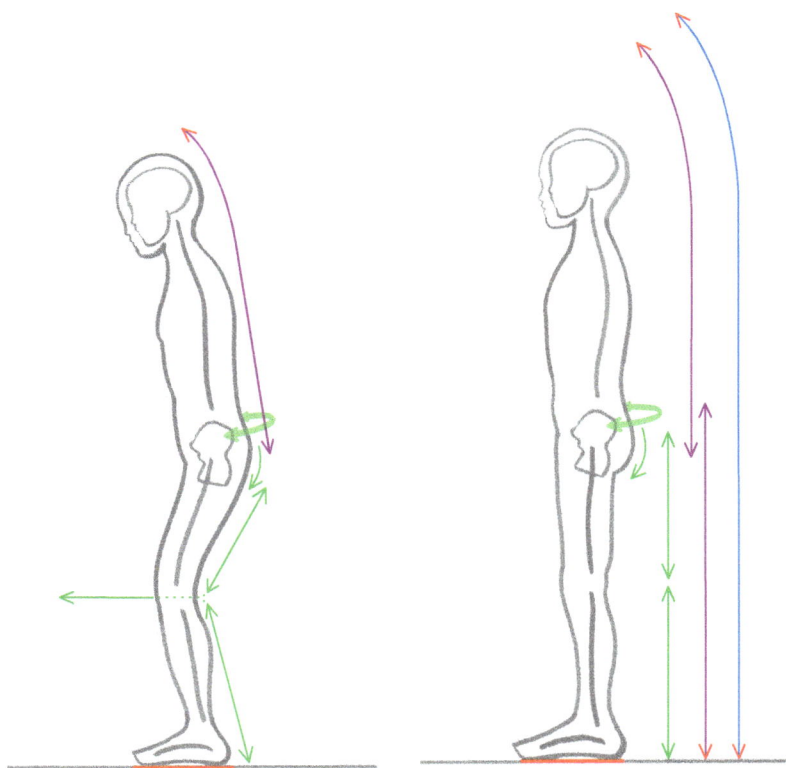

Breathing

All physical effort tends to increase thoracic rigidity.

F. MATTHIAS ALEXANDER[93]

Early in his career, FM was known as 'the breathing man'. This is no coincidence. His article 'The Theory and Practice of a New Method of Respiratory Re-education' was published in 1907.[94] FM came to the attention of the medical profession in connection with the help he was able to give patients with breathing. Many of FM's early pupils were actors, clergymen and orators, who were particularly interested in breathing and voice production.

Understanding breathing in the context of the primary control relationships is integral to a thorough understanding of our use and to working on ourselves.[95] Breathing is not an isolated function. It is inseparably connected to postural support, movement in general and emotional states. This connectedness points to the depth and circularity of the web of relationships that we summarise as the primary control. Any interference with the breath equally constitutes an interference to the effectiveness of the primary control relationships. Similarly, anything that reduces the freedom of our basic primary control relationships — neck, head, back, limbs and ground — adversely affects the freedom of the breath. And conversely, anything that frees the breath simultaneously supports primary control relationships that work more effectively (see Figure 1).

---

93 Alexander, *Universal Constant*, 43.
94 See F. Matthias Alexander, "The Theory and Practice of a New Method of Respiratory Re-education," in *Articles and Lectures*, ed. Jean M. Fischer (Mouritz, 2015), 53–71.
95 See 'Primary control relationships', page 11.

In all that follows, use your visual imagination: work with the pictures that I draw with words. We can start with the general assumption that more freedom—in you, me and all our pupils—is available. You are alive, so you are breathing and that means there is movement.

Exploration 9: What is moving?

This exploration is easiest while lying in semi-supine.[96] But the question 'what is moving?' can be asked in any position or situation. Your chest and abdomen probably move. This immediately means that your whole torso is involved. We know that the ribs can move sideways. As well for most of us, the abdomen comes out forwards a little as we breathe in. This is because all the internal organs are slightly displaced as air comes into the lungs and the ribs move out and the diaphragm descends. Any undue tension in the lower back or at the back of the waist may also contribute to movement at the boneless front, where there is the least resistance.

Start in semi-supine:

• Becoming quiet, open to what is, including your contact with your supporting surface;

• Refreshing an attitude of open, non-judgemental receptivity;

• Neutrally observing, as if from a distance, the fact that you are breathing; and

• All the while, quietly paying attention, remaining interested, without feeling things out, looking for sensation or rummaging.

You may observe

• Movement of the ribs sideways — this can include up under the armpits;

• Movement back and down and forward and up of the ends of the floating ribs;

• Slight rising of the chest; and

• Gentle displacement of all your abdominal contents.

Your abdomen is not just at the front, but also the sides and back (think of your waist). And the abdomen does not stop at your waist or belt line. It goes right to the floor of your pelvis. There may be a toning of the pelvic floor with the breath. In considering the abdomen, we need to include the full internal volume of the pelvis — vertically, side to side and front to back. That entire volume is available to you. FM talked about the floating ribs, but it may be more relatable to talk about your 'full circumference'. Remember: no rummaging!

96 This is simply because habits of postural support are not being triggered to the same extent when we are lying down as when we are upright. To the extent that there are poor habits in this regard, it means that when upright, you are supporting yourself with tension that interferes with the breath.

Exploration 10: What restricts your breath?

What might cause a restriction to your breath? Try any of the following, in semi-supine, sitting, standing or any other position. What effect does each have on your breath? Most people find that tension anywhere has a restricting effect on the breath. Give time in between each action to return to neutral, i.e., not tightening.

- Tightening your neck (this can extend muscularly to your shoulders, upper chest and upper back);
- Head going any version of 'in' (towards your neck or pelvis), not out;
- Narrowing anywhere;
- Tightening your buttocks;
- Tensing your pelvic floor;
- Stiffening your legs, feet or toes;
- Tightening your arms or hands; and
- Clenching your jaw.

Exploration 11: Identifying restrictions

Lie quietly in semi-supine, interested and watching with curiosity. It is usually apparent that your abdomen is gently rising and falling, as air goes in and out. Yet, of course, this abdominal movement is not that of the air itself moving. Rather, it represents the displacement of the viscera, as the shape of the chest cavity changes and the viscera are pressed upon by the descending diaphragm, when air comes in. When you are lying down, you need a minimal amount of air, so this movement is small. Yet while lying down, you still can quietly observe.[97]

As air comes in, you need to allow freedom both downwards (into the pelvis) and outwards (allowing the ribs to move). This is to ensure that abdominal tension or tension in the pelvic floor or leg attachments to the pelvis does not interfere with free displacement of your abdominal contents. The sides of your abdomen can elastically give, as can the back of your abdomen on either side of your spine (which will relate to the floating ribs) as well as the floor of your pelvis.[98]

If you pay attention to what you release on the in-breath, you realise that you must inadvertently be tightening these parts each time on the out-breath. Once you identify this, the job of working on yourself includes paying attention to not tightening these exact things on your exhale. So don't pull down on the exhale, and definitely don't go so far as to squeeze towards the end (or at any point earlier) of the exhale — squeezing might be most apparent in your legs, pelvic floor, lower back and front abdominal muscles. If you don't tighten them on the exhale, you won't have as much to release on the inhale. Note this also in the following exploration.

97   It may be of interest to see Frank H. Netter, "Variations in Position and Contour of Stomach in Relation to Body Habitus," in *Atlas of Human Anatomy* (ICON Learning Systems, 1997), plate 258. These are paintings of actual cadavers. How much are these different positions reflective of the use of the four different people? Do they suggest anything about each individual's breathing?

98   I do not want to encourage unnatural exaggeration of anything, including movement, in the abdomen. Rather, I want to bring to your attention something that is often missed, even by experienced teachers. We want the fullest freedom available in order to be responsive to whatever demands are made on the breath, whether they are being made or not, *and* in order to not interfere with the overall 'up'. It is very easy to restrict movement in the lower abdomen. That restriction generally seems to go with floating ribs that are not as free as they could be.

Exploration 12: Increasing the demand

Now we can increase the demand with a whispered ah, or any sibilant or vocalised sound. The first thing is to exhale — that way you have to inhale again. Think about the exhale, with the aim of not pulling down, shortening, squeezing, forcing or doing anything that exceeds balanced tone. A goal here is to move towards being able to differentiate between balanced tone and undue tension, while increasing demand, for example, a higher volume of sound. Working with a colleague who can monitor tone/tension can be helpful.

If you are working with whispered ahs, the sound you make on the exhale may tell you whether there are restrictions to the outflow of air and precisely what they may be. Each type of restriction has its own characteristic sound. Restrictions could include a depressed soft palate, a restriction at the back of the throat or a tight jaw. Any restriction represents a hindrance to the wished-for elasticity in your primary control relationships. FM expressed it this way: 'all "physical" tension tends to cause thoracic (chest) rigidity.'[99]

Then, release to allow air in:

- Not preventing the displacement of your abdominal contents: include releasing down (towards the pelvic floor) and allowing a filling/inhabiting of all of the volume of your pelvis. This is, of course, something that you picture in your mind's eye — it is not a felt doing.
- Allowing the ribs out sideways and releasing all the way around your circumference. Remember that your torso is three-dimensional. Consider the breadth and depth of your pelvis.

The release to allow air in can be an entirely seamless transition, not something sudden, jerky or tense-making. This is unlike what so many singers and wind or brass players practise, possibly due to mistakenly prioritising musical time constraints ahead of practising for freedom, or due to a lack of knowledge that it is possible to breathe otherwise.[100]

---

99   F. Matthias Alexander, *Constructive Conscious Control of the Individual* (Integral Press, 1955), 122.

100 See 'Exploration 14: Practising for freedom', page 94.

Exploration 13: Daily life

Any time you speak, see what you observe about your use with reference to your breath. If you happen to be a wind or brass player or singer, you have ample opportunity to watch what you do as you play or sing in the light of the previous exploration. You can use warmups or technical drills as vehicles for paying attention to your breath.

Exploration 14: Practising for freedom

Experiment with any of the explorations offered so far, while standing, sitting, moving about, semi-flexing, experiencing a stressful situation and so on. A primary goal is to cultivate the ability to breathe in freely.

- When you are standing, release up, right through your legs to the floor. As you inhale, have the intention for length/not to shorten down the back of your legs. To the extent that you tighten when breathing in, it will be observable in your legs — keep letting them go, particularly on the inhale!

Speed of inhalation is of particular relevance to singers, instrumentalists and actors. It develops as you learn to avoid unnecessary tightening. When practising, dispense with inhaling as governed by a metronome or the tempo of a piece. Take your time. It is about *practising for freedom*: freedom on the inhale and freedom on the exhale. If both are free, then you can raise the demand. For example, you can start to impose constraints like tempo, duration, volume or extremes of register. More demand may mean more muscular tone on the out-breath, which is fine. It is muscular. As you raise the demand, you can continue to use your self in a non-doing way, i.e., using muscular tone that is adequate to the task, with no pulling down. This means maintaining even, elastic tone throughout — not unduly tightening, for example, in your abdomen, neck, legs or pelvic floor.

Hand contact

The necessary foundations for hand contact and what it can convey lie in the primary control relationships and the corresponding coordinated elasticity. These are exemplified in semi-flexion, including attention to the ground and the breath. In the Alexander Technique, we are constantly zooming in for detail and stepping back again for a wider view. But ideally we keep both views simultaneously accessible. Now, we zoom in a little again, on the basis that as you consider your hands, you do not lose the wider picture of your use.

It's your whole nervous system

Your use of your self is the foundation for hands that have the sensitivity, delicacy and strength to convey a range of information, both in and out. Your hands are an extension of the rest of you. Here are some ways of framing the connections between your centre and your hands via your arms:

- There exist embryological connections between the scapulae/torso and arms/hands;
- FM's 'lifter' (back) muscles support the arms;
- The same conditions of use govern both freedom of the breath and support for the arms;
- We can recognise the connections between elastic breadth of the back, free breathing and support for the arms;
- We can allow length and breadth in the back to support the arms;
- We can let the elbows simultaneously release away from wrists and from shoulders, to create a clearer channel between the torso and the hands; and
- We can acknowledge the further connection from the floor through the legs and trunk to the arms and hands.

All of the preceding imply or can be expressed in any of the others, and they point to relevant directions.

Keep some version of these directions in mind as you play with the following explorations. Be curious about where greater freedom may be available, including in your hands, or further back (proximally) from your hands: in your arms, shoulders, torso/back or via attending to your breath. There are too many possible ways of interrupting freedom to provide preventive directions for them all here.

Working with your hands supinated and hands pronated (palm up or palm down) and thinking about the differences that arise between the two orientations may illuminate some useful points—consider anything you need to include to work on yourself. I assume that you continue to pay attention to all your basic directions, and that these remain primary as you go through the following explorations.

Exploration 15: Palm contact and hands supine

Sit with your palms resting on your thighs (i.e., hands pronated) reasonably close to your torso, such that your arms do not pull on your shoulders. There should be no strain or effort in this position. The contact for your palms is helpful for what follows. The palm contact is a source of information for your nervous system about how it can organise you in space, like your bottom on a chair or your feet on the floor. This is also relevant when you put your hands on someone else.

Now ask for length and breadth in your hands: breadth across the palms, importantly including the heels of the palms (from the base of the thumbs to the ulnar edge) and length all the way through to the fingertips. Check your wrists, asking for breadth and depth between the outside and palm side (from dorsal to palmar). Can you let your elbows hang freely from your shoulders while maintaining the support for your shoulders from your back as a whole? That is, can your arms be energised yet not heavy? Think also of the opposition between your elbows and wrists.

All this assumes and rests on your background intent for all the basics: not to tighten your neck, not to pull back your head, and allowing length and width throughout your back. Another way of working is to bring attention to your primary contact points — sitting bones and feet, along with your visual contact with the space you are in — while allowing freedom for the breath to move, with an intention for length and volume throughout your torso.

Then, gently and thoughtfully turn your hands over (i.e., hands supinated) and go through the preceding sequence again. What you need to attend to may change depending on whether your hands are pronated or supinated.

Exploration 16: Prayer position v1

While sitting, standing or lying down, bring your palms together, fingers pointing upwards, as in a prayer position. Start with renewing the idea of your shoulders and arms being supported from around the bottom of your back and the back of your waist. Then ask for both length and breadth in your hands: breadth across the palms, including the heels of the palms (from the base of the thumbs to the ulnar edge) and length all the way through to the fingertips. Check your wrists, asking for breadth and depth through from the palm side to the outside (palmar to dorsal). Can you let your elbows hang freely from your shoulders while maintaining the support for your shoulders from your back as a whole? Is there freedom in the upper parts of your upper arms (or are you pulling in across the fronts of your armpits)?

Exploration 17: Prayer position v2

Move your prayer-position hands while maintaining the hand-to-hand contact, for example, to the left, right, up, down, closer to you and further away. Continue to apply all the checkpoints and directions from the previous two explorations.

Exploration 18: Prayer position v3

Stand sideways in a doorway. Again, use prayer-position hands. But this time, place your hands on either side of the wall whose edge you face, while you move sideways, first one way, then the other, in the doorway. You can also try getting lower or higher — use semi-flexion or go up onto your toes. Still apply all the considerations from the preceding explorations.

All of these (Explorations 15–18) can be explored with a partner's hands monitoring you. Alternatively, instead of having your own hands together, have contact with your partner's hands.

Exploration 19: Hands and rocking on all fours

The following comments about all fours are not intended to be comprehensive but rather to offer some suggestions to those who wish to experiment.

Remember that your hands are the end of a whole system. For the hands to be alive and elastic, so too must be the rest of you.

In the matter of encouraging openness of the hands, working on all fours, both rocking and crawling, can be useful. You can experiment with your fingers splayed or together. In either case, a key point is to not collapse through the shoulders and arms onto the hands. It should not feel like your hands are carrying an undue weight. Your hands may be directly under your shoulders, or if your wrists object to this, have your hands further forward.

> Use the hand contacts to expand up off, with your whole torso toning, rather than collapsing between your arms and legs, or otherwise fixing. Also, don't collapse between your scapulae. Note that width across your back — including between the scapulae, with the ribs supporting them while allowed to freely move with the breath — provides support. Your whole torso can spring, through your arms and your legs, off the contacts that you have with the floor, principally via your hands and knees. Your head is still prepared to lead, your back can continue to lengthen and widen, and your three-dimensional torso continues to be breathed, from the base of your skull to the base of your pelvis.
>
> All of the foregoing takes time to read and think through. Yet, particularly when beginning to work on all fours, you should not remain still for long — gentle movement is desirable to facilitate working through the foregoing directions. Begin by rocking backwards, having noted where you are in space over your hands to start. You do not need to come further forward than your starting point as you rock, to minimise wrist strain. Pay due attention to your head direction, along with maintaining tone in your arms (don't lock your elbows), your three-dimensional torso toning up off your hands and knees, while releasing your legs. In particular, think about releasing around your bottom, the backs of your thighs and calves. If these directions are new to you, it can take a few weeks to put them all together.[101]

101 See 'Exploration 2: All fours', page 72.

Exploration 20: Hands and crawling

Still leading with your head and starting with a front limb, i.e., an arm, take all fours into a gentle crawling movement. Let your feet (dorsal surfaces) remain in contact with the floor, i.e., don't lift them but let them drag; same for the knees. The knees swing forwards enough to not be left behind, but not so much that they propel you — the head leads.

Hands on the back of a chair

Hands on the back of a chair is usually a training course exercise. It involves using inhibition and direction to train us in all the elements we need for the acquisition and ongoing development of hands-on skills. The non-doing, yet clear, well-directed contact that we want to give our pupil depends upon these skills.

Why use this apparently arcane form? Working with hands on the back of a chair should make clear that using your hands means attending to your use as a whole. This procedure involves not just your hands but, like all of Alexander's procedures, your whole body, the quality of your attention and the extent of your inhibition, i.e., the use of your self. It is about cultivating an overall elastic, toned expansion throughout, all while applying your hands. You refine the use of toned, energised hands without undue tension in your hands or anywhere else.[102] This builds your ability to become an open, elastic conduit between the floor and what your hands touch.

---

102 This lines up with the idea of 'non-doing doing'. As one becomes more experienced, using relatively active guidance with the hands when teaching may sometimes seem appropriate. The ability to do this effectively rests on your ability to maintain your overall elastic expansion/clear oppositional pulls.

Form and elasticity

The hands on the back of a chair form starts with semi-flexion.[103] This should bring an overall gravity-related, toned elasticity, encompassing a free neck, head going forward and out, back lengthening and widening, and free legs, i.e., an open channel between floor and hands. Then we add the hands on the back rail of the chair, without losing any of the foregoing. There are many ways of going wrong when we add the arms and hands. However, in general, we want to avoid anything that interferes with a free neck; we want free arms and wrists; we want the back to continue to support full and free breathing; and we want legs that remain elastic and free, open conduits to the floor contact. Without freedom in the legs, the hands are more constrained. Coordinating the various elements, each challenging on its own, usually requires careful building up before it can be effectively put together. The discussion and explorations given next break down the hands on the back of a chair procedure into smaller progressions. When these smaller pieces are familiar, you can put them together with standing semi-flexion.

The form for hands on the back of a chair—semi-flexion with a particular hand and arm position—is one thing, but getting real expansion is another.[104] Often, what gets practised is only the form, which is certainly not a waste of time. However, the practice of this procedure offers a gold mine, and stopping at the form means you may get some gold dust but you will miss out on the big nuggets—an overall toned, gravity-related, elastic expansion that includes both the arms and legs. This is what creates sensitive hands that can communicate.

---

103   See 'Semi-flexion', page 59.
104   See the anecdote in 'Is it actually semi-flexion?', page 61.

Exploration 21: Hand position for hands on the back of a chair

The unfamiliarity of the hand position may be challenging. You can play with this while sitting or sitting semi–flexed (torso angled forward), and with one hand at a time. This is about active, toned use of your hands and their delivery system (the arms and their connections), while maintaining all the basic relationships (not tightening your neck, back, breath or chair/floor contact). Build the elements individually before bringing them together, yet always keeping in mind the whole of you, without sacrificing any one element for any of the others.

- Bring one hand up so that your forearm is approximately horizontal. The palm faces down and your fingers are extended gently. Then fold straight fingers at the knuckles to approximately 90 degrees. Swing your extended thumb around to oppose your straight forefinger. Do not raise (flex) your wrist. You may need to attend to letting your wrist drop, as you slide your thumb down a little to oppose the forefinger;

- Now repeat with the other hand;

- Let your elbows lengthen away from your wrists, while they also release out of both the backs and fronts of your shoulders;

- Let your wrists widen and deepen;

- Allow your legs to be free (applies to both sitting and standing); and

- Continue to direct your neck, head and back (three–dimensional torso).

Pitfalls include locking the thumb, narrowing across the heel of the hand, tightening in the wrists or elbows, fixing the shoulders, holding the breath, tightening contact with the chair or floor, gripping the tongue or jaw and so on. Note that maintaining your good use trumps 'correct hand position', which remains aspirational. Your intent must not flip over into a doing.

Practice of this should help you develop hands which are neither too 'do–y' nor ineffectual and energy–less.[105]

---

105 'Another kind of badly' would be to use your hands on a pupil without energy or direction. Such a way of working might be acceptable—not intrusive—for the pupil, but is unlikely to be interesting or convey integration. This energy–less, ineffectual way of working often represents a misunderstanding of the meaning of 'non-doing'. Non-doing is not the absence of activity. It means having all oppositions active, which implies the absence of *unnecessary* tightening.

Exploration 22: Sitting semi-flexion

It can be useful to rehearse sitting semi-flexion. This is because if we include the complexities of standing semi-flexion, there may be too much to juggle at the level of skill we aspire to.[106]

- Start seated, with your torso upright. Note your sitting bones and give time to release your buttocks, legs and breath;
- Then rock gently forward *just a little*, and pause to give time to release your buttocks, legs and breath;
- Then rock back to your starting point, again giving time to release your buttocks, legs and breath; and
- Repeat slowly enough to get used to putting these directions together.

This simple forward and back movement usually takes a little practice to manage without tightening your buttocks or legs or holding your breath. It is a useful directed activity on its own. But I also offer it here because it provides a basis for what follows, both sitting and standing.

---

106 See "Illustration," in Alexander, *Constructive Conscious Control*, 108.

Exploration 23: Sitting semi-flexion to hands on the back of a chair

- Seated, with a suitable chair placed in front of you, bring one hand up onto its back rail, folding straight fingers at the knuckles and opposing your forefinger with your thumb. Do not raise (flex) your wrists. You may need to attend to letting your wrists drop, as you slide your thumb down the back rail of the chair to oppose the forefinger. You may need to rock forward on your sitting bones so that your torso/shoulder/arm/hand coordination can be optimal to the task.
- Repeat with the other hand so you have both hands on.

Pitfalls include locking the thumb, narrowing across the heel of the hand, tightening in the wrists or elbows, fixing the shoulders, holding the breath, tightening contact with the chair or floor, gripping the tongue or jaw and so on. Note that maintaining your good use trumps 'correct hand position', which remains aspirational. Your intent must not flip over into a doing.

While maintaining the tone in your fingers and hands,

- Let your elbows lengthen away from your wrists, while they also release out of both the backs and fronts of your shoulders. Your elbows should be able to be freely moved by someone else;
- Let your wrists widen and deepen;
- Allow your legs to be free (applies to both sitting and standing); and
- Continue to direct your neck, head and back (three-dimensional torso).

Once you can juggle these directions when sitting, revise your elastic standing semi-flexion. Then, move to the next exploration.

Exploration 24: Standing semi-flexion to hands on the back of a chair v1

From standing semi-flexion, place your hands on the back rail of a chair as described in Exploration 23. Again, don't compromise your general elasticity, particularly in the arms, the breath to the pelvic floor, the floor contact or freedom of the neck.

You need a firm but gentle hold of the back rail. To challenge your ability to not lose your overall elasticity anywhere, you can try a firmer grip.

Exploration 25: Standing semi-flexion to hands on the back of a chair v2

If you want to raise the demand further still, while maintaining your 'firm but gentle' grip, pull sideways on the back rail of the chair as if you want to make it longer (i.e., hands away from each other). Crucially, maintain the same elastic conditions in yourself. If you can pull on the back rail and not tighten — but rather continue your oppositional, toned elasticity, which equates to freedom in the breath and grounded lightness — you can also apply this same quality in the use of your hands on a person. If you already find this is easy, you have either done lots of work on yourself, or you may be missing something!

Summary

In semi-flexion and when practising hands on the back of a chair:

· Intend forward and upward freedom along your spine to your head;

· Intend length and width throughout your back;

· Allow your legs to be toned and responsive to the ground contact;

· Let your arms extend from your lengthening/widening/ breathing torso;

· Energise through to your fingertips without stiffening your fingers;

· Point your free elbows away from your wrists, and don't get hooked up in your shoulders; and

· Allow freedom for the breath — availability of the floating ribs and the volume of your pelvis as well as of your chest.

...all of which belong to the working of the primary control.

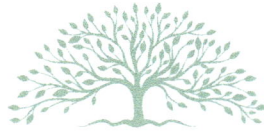

CHAPTER 5

The teaching journey— A lifelong exploration

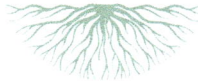

La ruta nos aportó otro paso natural. (The path itself brings forth for us the natural next step.)

OLD SPANISH SAYING

Practising

When he was 81, Pablo Casals, the greatest cellist of the twentieth century, was asked why he continued to practise daily. He replied, 'Because I think I am making progress.'[107]

It is clear from those who knew him that Alexander's skills became more refined over his lifetime. You can't get good at something if you don't practise it. To develop the skills to become a teacher of the Alexander Technique involves a process of working on the use of your self. To develop as a teacher, you have to continue working on your self as you teach.

---

107 *A Day in the Life of Pablo Casals* (film), directed by Robert Snyder (1957).

In the process of working on your own use of your self as a pupil, a trainee teacher and beyond, you probably have had one transformative experience after another—moments of insight and understanding. Your teaching is informed by these experiences: they are part of what you bring to each lesson. Yet each experience is yours only. And each experience is about the process—inhibition and direction applied in a particular context—not about the experience itself.

While being kind to yourself, yet not complacent, self-enquiry can help you continue to clarify the what, why and how of teaching. The ongoing evolution into greater competence can be fed by asking yourself questions such as

- What am I teaching?
- What do I want my pupils to learn?
- Why teach this way and not that?
- Why teach in this order and not that?
- Why am I putting my hands on here rather than there?
- Why am I using my hands at all? What do I want to achieve?
- How can I communicate better? How do I communicate verbally?
- How do others do this, and can I learn from them?
- How do I recognise and attach meaning to what I perceive with my hands?

Answers to these questions may not be immediate, and they may change with time; the value lies in asking, since the answers may require thoughtfulness and attentiveness. Any answers still leave an abundance of freedom for each individual teacher in how they teach.

Hands, embodiment, repetition and attention

Over the years, pupils have sometimes commented on my 'healing hands'. I always reply that whatever I am doing is not mysterious. It is an entirely learned skill.

Using the hands in teaching is a consciously cultivated skill arising out of a practice, that of paying attention to yourself with reference to your primary control relationships, with interested, non-doing curiosity. You cultivate an attitude of quiet, and with some idea—usually conveyed by your teachers—of a blueprint of possibilities. On graduating as an Alexander Technique teacher, this learned skill should be adequate to begin teaching. And hopefully you are inspired by your teachers to continue using the tools learnt during formal training to work on yourself with a completely open-ended attitude.[108]

With hands-on work, it is important to remember that, while putting your hands on a pupil is an obvious element in teaching, it is the very last step of your own process. This process is anything but apparent. There is a particular quality of touch that you seek to develop through working on yourself. It invites the person being touched to expand in some way—physically, in their awareness, in their attentiveness or their mental or emotional horizon. Our touch depends on our ability to be a conduit for quiet. Cultivating this ability takes

---

108 There may be a valid comparison with the maturing of a musician. For deepening development over time, the musician needs to continue to listen attentively to themselves, with the expectation of incremental improvement, probably imperceptible from one day to the next. It is implicit that the musician aims for all available refinement every time they play, listening (paying attention) and thus constantly using the basic skills or building blocks to extend themselves a little further. It is not the instrument that sounds good but the musician who plays it.

time. When you touch someone, you communicate something of your own coordination, something of the state of your own nervous system. For your touch to not be unpleasant, let alone for your hands to be sensitive to the person you are touching and to be able to communicate something about the Alexander Technique, i.e., inhibition and direction, you have to spend time improving your own use. This means paying attention to yourself and refining the steering of your own nervous system. The use of the hands in Alexander Technique teaching is not so much about the use of the hands as it is about the use of the self. The quality of your touch is a function of your whole self.[109]

Before we can hope to teach anyone about the Alexander Technique, we must ourselves embody and exemplify what we want to teach, through our own practice and application of it. We have to have gone through the process of learning how to work effectively on ourselves. Then we need to be able to communicate this process, and deliver it progressively so that a pupil or class can take it in. The key concepts—use, primary control, inhibition and direction—need to be communicated, but we don't need to get stuck on the particular, traditionally used jargon words. What is more important is the meanings of the words. We want to help our pupils gain the practical experience that corresponds to the words, and to internalise their meanings. We don't want mystery: we want understanding. Understanding is empowering. Above all else, a teacher's job, whether they are teaching the Alexander Technique or anything else, is to empower people to learn for themselves.

As teachers, we aspire to embodying inhibition—a state of being available to stimuli, outer and inner, without looking for inputs and without grabbing or judging them as they

---

109   See 'Hand contact', page 95.

arrive, i.e., without undue reactivity. Nor do we want to follow thoughts, sensations or feelings into daydreaming, but rather to allow authentic, reasoned responses to the present moment. As trainees or Alexander Technique teachers, we want to continue to apply 'man's supreme inheritance of conscious guidance and control'[110] — to be able to respond to life's little and big stimuli by choosing to become more alive, responsive and elastic, not less. And when faced with a pupil, the same applies, only more so. We must, therefore, practise our aspiration to respond to life with inhibition and direction, giving ourselves time and space. Happily, everything can become a vehicle for our practice. This certainly includes when we are refining our elasticity in cultivating our hands. We need to let go of expectations, judging, seeking, rummaging, poking about or feeling something out. Be patient and forgiving, and let go of any need to understand immediately. Be inquisitive and stick to principle — remember AR's cauliflower.[111]

In everyday life, working with inhibition and direction is a practice of mindful, embodied attention. Like any practice, applying the Alexander Technique appears repetitive. You must endlessly follow process: paying attention, inhibiting and directing. You repeat procedures, working at your practice of attentiveness. With the right sort of repetition comes a gradual deepening of your understanding, both kinaesthetically and intellectually. Contrarily, in fact, you want never to actually repeat yourself — that would be counterproductive and boring. It is rather a case of practising 'beginner's mind'.[112]

---

110 Alexander, *Man's Supreme Inheritance*, 137.
111 'Be patient, stick to principle and it will all open up like a great cauliflower.' AR Alexander on how to learn the Alexander Technique, quoted in Jones, *Body Awareness*, 68.
112 See Shunryu Suzuki, *Zen Mind, Beginner's Mind* (Shambhala, 2006).

You may aspire to one hundred percent attentiveness, while recognising that the approach is to accept at any moment just a little more attentiveness than whenever you started. The point is to be moving in the right direction, however slowly. You start by renewing your intent to pay attention and be interested, staying fresh and not repeating. It is a process of refreshing your intentions, over and over. Thus, you cultivate the *habit of attentiveness*.

Expectations and aspirations

It is reasonable to have an expectation of gradual, steady, ongoing improvement in our use or in the development of teaching skills. We can have a clear aspiration without being attached to achieving it in a particular timeframe. We might describe aspiration as an intention without attachment to an immediate outcome, underpinned by the means; an attitude of optimising our manner of use as an immediate way of life. Inhibition exists in relation to aspirations or goals. If FM had had no goal motivating him, we might not have the Alexander Technique today. And as already noted, FM's hand skills improved over the course of his life.

As a trainee or new teacher, you work on your manual teaching skills using inhibition applied to a range of procedures or directed activities. It makes sense to approach the practice with an attitude of quality over quantity. When you invest time in working on a skill, it is vital to not be in a hurry. You don't want to practise performing at a level below that which you are capable of. Remember that your hands-on skills are the end of a sequence and that there are no shortcuts to the process. Every time you use your hands in teaching, it is an opportunity to practise inhibition: quality over quantity, not hurrying but rather producing your non-doing, attentive, detached best.

In teachers, ideally some degree of 'up' is ticking away all the time. Over time, conscious, deliberate preparation establishes an ever more positive *manner* of use, and more gradually, improvement in *conditions* of use, available in response to whatever we are faced with.

As a new teacher, I continued taking semi-regular lessons from more experienced teachers for some years because it was clear that this input was helpful. I was learning. In between lessons, I would work with that learning. This typically included going over hands on the back of a chair for a few minutes each morning in my teaching room, ahead of starting my own teaching day. This woke up my thinking and fine-tuned my process of directing. By the time I greeted the day's first pupil, I would be reliably going 'up'. Each lesson I then gave was, equally, time spent continuing to refine my own use. Eventually, just the act of walking into my teaching room triggered a positive change, towards the higher end of my use spectrum. This was, I believe, a consequence of practising the application of inhibition and direction using the vehicles of hands on the back of a chair, whispered ahs and other procedures, as well as paying attention to my use in general. Gradually, I was becoming more sensitive to information coming in and clearer with information going out.

Discipline and will

To pay attention in the way I have been describing, and to apply the Alexander Technique in life, is an act of will. Invariably, in continuing to work on yourself, what triggers a smaller or bigger lightbulb to turn on is some realisation, experience or sensation. It is probably something new that has come into focus. Perhaps you have just let go of something that you hadn't noticed before or that somehow was not previously available to you to control. This experience alerts you to something that you can be awake to in yourself as you go through your day. Examples are almost endless. Physically, you might realise that you needlessly hang on to your jaw or to your tongue. You might notice, if you think about it, that you have the capacity to release your ankles or the backs of your legs more, and when you do, this leads to a better connection to the ground. Or you might recognise something about the nature of your reactions—in general or to a particular emotional need. While these examples may have significance, they are possibly trivial in comparison to what they represent: the opportunity for exercising your will in choosing to inhibit and direct, over and over. You can make it new every time.

You may have been working on yourself in this way already, perhaps for many years. It just continues.[113] As you come back to yourself again and again, with non-judgemental attentiveness, you steadily internalise any particular new awareness. With each refinement, you render yourself more sensitive to your own manner of use. This is necessary to becoming more sensitive to someone else's use. It is how you go from taking care of yourself to sensing the other: by practising an attitude of receptivity, one of being interested and finding out, not crashing in with your mind already made up (more of AR's cauliflower). It also requires the ability to make yourself a springy, elastic conduit between the floor and your hands. It takes time to start to perceive with your hands, and to develop an understanding of what you are perceiving. The means of developing the skill of perception are exactly the same as those for developing the skill of using your hands at all, in a non-coercive, non-doing, non-end-gaining way. Learning to put your hands on someone out of your own grounded

---

113 See 'Inhibition and sensation', page 20.

elasticity means you simultaneously learn the conditions for perception. This is not something that can be forced: it does itself, over time, in some proportion to your ability to inhibit.

If you are attentive enough to use your self at the upper end of what you are capable of, this upper end becomes your new norm and a higher upper end becomes correspondingly available.[114] You continue to make your best into your norm. This is a continuous and open-ended process, as you move along the spectrum of your evolving use. Underlying all this is an attitude of open attentiveness, interest and curiosity, and the assumption that maybe there's more. Other useful qualities in this endeavour include humility and persistence. Keeping a reflective diary where you note new insights or discoveries can be a helpful practice.

Teaching notes

Teaching anything involves many elements. Some of the elements relevant to teaching the Alexander Technique include understanding how to make each lesson a positive experience for the pupil, dealing with our own and our pupil's personal space, clarifying what we want to achieve with our hands and how we use words, the use of stories, the role of sensation, and understanding what makes the Alexander Technique different.

---

114 Cardiovascular fitness may provide a good analogy. After a bout of ill health, I returned to exercise over a period of several weeks. I started with a gentle ten-minute walk. Then, I gradually raised the demand, walking a little further, including a small hill, then a larger hill, eventually breaking into a light jog-trot and so on. I consciously underdid the demand each time, staying well within my comfort zone, while still doing a little more. After six months, I was nearly back to full fitness i.e., with good use. I always operated within the zone of what I was capable of managing well, and importantly, at the upper end of that zone. Thus, my zone of capacity steadily extended.

What is teaching (not)?

My colleague, Amanda,[115] is a fine teacher of the Alexander Technique. Before Alexander, she studied the piano. A more than competent amateur, in her youth she performed concerti with her local orchestra. She still practises daily. From time to time, she has sought out a piano teacher for inspiration, coaching and to maintain momentum in her musical journey. In one instance, a local piano teacher came highly recommended. Incidentally, Amanda had given Alexander Technique lessons to a number of this teacher's pupils. Amanda arranged to see the teacher with a view to the possibility of regular piano lessons.

At the much-anticipated lesson, the teacher did not appear interested in why Amanda had sought her out, nor what she was interested in getting out of the lesson. There was no acknowledgement at all of her, no establishing of a connection. The piano teacher was, however, endlessly keen to convey something about a particular element of piano technique that did not seem to have any relevance at that point. Or if it did, the teacher failed to make the relevance clear. She demonstrated the technique, yet offered nothing comprehensible as to why or how, and conspicuously did not change tack when it was clear that Amanda was not relating to her approach.

It was a wonderful demonstration of how not to teach. Amanda left the lesson feeling that she had not been met or seen. The interaction was all about the teacher and not at all about the pupil. The teacher had not inspired, enthused, encouraged, empowered or inculcated any aspiration in her pupil.

---

115   This is a pseudonym.

In contrast to this story, you

· Need to listen;

· Can meet the pupil where they are, every time;

· Can cultivate qualities displayed by good teachers: curiosity, humility, courage and persistence;

· Can be confident, yet always assume that you don't know everything;

· Want to help your pupil build their tools for self-work;

· Want to inspire your pupil and show them how to aspire; and

· Can keep asking yourself, 'What does this person need to know?' and 'What information are they missing?'

Teach your pupil what they can grasp or influence — empower your pupil. If you tell them about something that they can't do anything about, you do not empower them. Three fundamentals you can seek to convey in a single lesson and over a course of lessons are

· That use affects functioning;

· The pupil's agency; and

· Anatomical points of orientation (mapping) to help the pupil understand the first two items.

Qualities to bring into the teaching room

Qualities to cultivate include calm, energy, enthusiasm, openness (to what might happen or what you may learn), expansiveness and empathy. Being accepting and non-judgemental, showing interest in your pupil, including in how you physically approach them, are basic.

In considering desirable qualities, we can also highlight some dangers of being an Alexander teacher. These include overconfidence, certainty and even arrogance—anything that makes you assume that your understanding of your pupil's problem, or even your understanding of the Alexander Technique, is complete. It's okay to say, 'I don't know,' 'I'm not sure' or 'This is outside of my area of expertise.' Assume that you can always learn and that you can learn something from anyone, including your pupils. There are always things that you don't know or that you could miss.

Personal space

Every time you are close enough to put hands on a pupil, you are in their personal space. Recognise and acknowledge your own space as well as theirs, as part of your attitude to physically approaching your pupil. Your pre-hands-on checklist may be some version of this:

- Free my neck (head–torso relationship);
- Back to lengthen and widen (length with breadth and with depth from the base of my pelvis to the base of my skull)—let my back be breathed;
- Acknowledge contact with the ground (allow weight through my bones to the floor, allow the floor up through my legs); and
- Respect the pupil's personal space and be aware of my own.

In all this, aspire for your attention to include both you and your pupil. And you still come first.

Hands

We want our hands to be able to convey

- Acceptance: non-judgemental, listening hands that don't ask for anything are trusted;
- Empowerment for the pupil to think for themselves, as opposed to the teacher overdoing or underdoing;
- How to 'see' or 'think' a part of the body;
- The possibility of change;
- Guidance with spatial direction;
- Support for all of the foregoing;
- An open attitude of 'I don't know,' giving the pupil space to find their own knowing;
- A contact or reference point, a point of interest or curiosity;
- Calm; and
- How to recognise sensation without needing to go into it.

With our hands, we can encourage an alive, energised, elastic, coordinated relationship of the different parts of the body, one to another. Ideally, we aspire to an ever more sensitive, tactile 'conversation' with our pupil, the content of which is inhibition and direction, accompanied by appropriate and timely verbal explanations and instructions.

When you use your hands, you want to be able to ask yourself

- Is my pupil going 'up' or 'down', and how strongly?
- If they are going down, what do they need to stop doing, and how?
- How can they achieve greater integration?
- What is amenable right now to some sort of positive change?
- What can I help the pupil change, and in what order (as opposed to moving bits about, 'fixing' a shape etc.)?

- What words would be helpful for my pupil to hear?
- Is my pupil's mental picture of their physicality accurate?
- If not, how can my pupil amend their way of seeing themselves to render the messages flooding their neuro-musculature more accurate?
- Where do I start in the process of helping my pupil to simplify their pattern of use?
- How best can I convey this possibility?

You as the teacher use your hands to reflect, respond to and guide the pupil's understanding of possibilities, i.e., possibilities of new or unfamiliar relationships and directions. Such a two-way conversation cannot be forced. It is a sophisticated and disciplined ability that takes time to cultivate.

Hands may be augmented with words to convey the simult-aneity and interdependence of primary control relationships. For example, you want to indicate to your pupil something about not locking their knees back, while you have a hand on their neck. That hand will be communicating 'don't tighten here' (the neck). It might also be asking for length down the back. (Or you might have both of your hands on their ribs at the back to a similar effect.) The hands are giving a clear non-verbal reminder of up or decompression as, simultaneously, you give the additional verbal instruction about the knees. In this way, you can help your pupil learn to juggle multiple directions; connect a freer neck with unlocked knees and a lengthening back, and build a connected sequence of directions.

Words

There is an art to keeping meaningful communication going between you and your pupil. It can encompass steadily bringing out the need for your pupil's participation and its nature, as well as being alive to opportunities to illuminate teaching points.

What does the pupil need to hear? Aim for minimum words and maximum clarity. Say what you mean as concisely as possible. Your message can get lost or confused if you use too many words. We need to convey meaning, not teach jargon. Indeed, the meaning we want to convey is more important than the words we use. We need to remain crystal clear about what we are teaching, including the why and the how as well as their sequence. If you find yourself talking a lot, this may be a warning signal that you have got lost in theory. Teaching the Alexander Technique is never about external knowledge—you need to make it immediate and practical. Sometimes, words can be helpful distractions for your pupil, for example, if they are trying too hard, or else disappearing into feeling out their sensations. Equally, don't be afraid of silence—reducing the level of stimulation can be constructive.

With each pupil or group, you gradually build a common language which relates to their use. Generally, language needs to be definite and specific, not vague. Be conscious that choosing your words is a part of good teaching. Your pupil needs to know what you mean by any given word or phrase. Often, your hands will deliver the meaning. Initially, it's your hands that provide the important guidance. For example, using certain words or conveying a specific idea and simultaneously touching somewhere in particular can connect your terminology with the pupil's experience, which they can start to comprehend through the words. For example, consider a pupil who habitually tenses their lower back or legs. As you say something like, 'Allow widening across your lower back' or 'Invite "give" across the back of your pelvis,' you place your directed hand on the pupil's lower back or on the back of the pupil's pelvis. Your pupil eventually starts to allow this widening, and you confirm to them that this is what you want. You reiterate this a number of times, probably over several lessons, repeatedly giving your pupil the opportunity to practise sending their directions. You possibly point out associated undoing—say, in their legs or their breathing. Gradually, the pupil develops the capacity to use just your hand contact to trigger the requisite release (meaning they have internalised their directions), and they have words with which they can describe the process. Eventually, just tapping a finger at the back of your pupil's pelvis may not only remind the pupil of their newly developed direction to allow the widening, but also of the whole sequence of associated directions, if you have been making these connections clear. In this example, they might free their legs or their breath as their lower back releases. Your words, initially an undefined clue, have acquired precise, practical meaning.

Principles can be demonstrated all the way through a lesson. Use every opportunity to anchor your pupil's experience to the principles, and refer to them. Yet, while teaching about inhibition, direction, use, primary control relationships, faulty sensory appreciation, habit or non-doing, you may choose to not name them until after the pupil has started to have clear experiences of their meaning. This underlines that the actual word, for example, inhibition, may be less important than its attached meaning. What is the meaning you aspire to when you use the words? Recognise that the experience defines the words. The words follow the experience; they are a wonderful checklist and they may describe what success will look like. But they are symbols, not the meaning or condition itself.

It is always possible to find something positive to say to your pupil. Acknowledge and validate what is going well. Steer your pupil gently, ideally so gently that they don't even know they are being steered. Find forms of words that encourage. For instance, instead of saying, 'You are still tightening' try 'Can you allow this to be even freer?' Make no value judgements in your comments such as, 'Wow, this is tight' or 'Yep, that massage therapist was right about your neck.' Rather, acknowledge when there is any improvement in the 'wrong' thing, from your point of view. Point out your pupil's agency in their change—offer encouragement and empowerment. Convey the idea that if they give it a little attention, they can make the change their own—foster aspiration. Make this immediate, pointing out when your pupil has an experience of greater ease or integration that it was something in which they had agency.

Stay on message—if your pupil leaves the lesson with one new idea to work with, you have done your job. Build concepts gradually, reinforcing basic principles. Use repetition that doesn't seem like repetition—lots of different ways of conveying the same thing. Straight repetition eventually ceases to be alive; our brains respond to change. For example, find multiple ways of saying 'release', like unclench, undo, relax, un-grip or soften. There may be several ways of highlighting a particular point. For example, 'pulling your head back and down', 'scrunching your neck', 'pulling your head in' or 'unnecessarily involving your neck muscles' is 'unhelpful', 'misplaced', 'unnecessary' or 'doesn't belong to the situation'. You can add why this is so and the implications of not making a change.

In any case, the more ways you can express an idea, the more likely you are to find words that your pupil can relate to.

Edit what you say (don't speak for too long), find a through-line, a logical sequence in the lesson and relate it to your pupil's experience. Pick up on cues (often verbal) from your pupil. Use and build on their own words, language and images. For instance, your pupil may say that their head feels like it's floating like a buoy on water. You may interpret this as a positive experience of a freer neck or greater freedom in general. Then, you could add the picture of a buoy needing an anchor lest it float away—the image and maybe your pupil need some sort of grounding.

While speaking, pay attention to the speed of your delivery. Listen to the sound of your own voice. Your pupil needs to be able to keep up, so don't speak too fast. Sometimes you need to deliberately slow your delivery, or speak more loudly or clearly. Indicators may include that your pupil uses hearing aids; you are not communicating in your pupil's first language; you are teaching in an echoey room or you have a pupil who struggles with the new ideas. Take your time, and remember you don't have to talk the whole time; your hands are a constant conduit and they are speaking to the whole pupil, not just to the bit you are touching.

On the other side, if your pupil talks too much and doesn't pay due attention, you may choose to interrupt: 'I want to hear what you have to tell me, but for the moment, come back to what's happening right now.' You might then put your hand where you think they need to pay attention, for example, on their neck or lower back, and ask them to give attention there. Then, having brought your pupil back to themselves, chances are they will fall silent as they pay attention. But if they don't redirect their attention, you may keep bringing them back to whatever needs their attention, over and over.

In all this, remember the acronym KIS—keep it simple! Avoid jargon, keep it practical and relate the lesson to your pupil's life.

Stories

Humans learn and remember through stories. We can teach using stories. It is possible to illustrate almost any learning or teaching point with a story. This applies equally in one-to-one lessons or in groups. Here is the story of how I started with the Alexander Technique. Without naming them, I touch on various Alexandrian ideas, including use, end-gaining, the means whereby, faulty sensory appreciation and the notion that the Alexander Technique might be able to address problems that other knowledge frameworks cannot.

After high school, I studied at the New South Wales State Conservatorium of Music in Sydney.[116] I practised my instrument, the trombone, diligently and I was also working full time in a professional orchestra. Thus, I played a great deal, every day. I was getting positive strokes for my hard work, but I had no idea that I was 'overdoing'. The excessive tension and effort that I used in playing (and living) at the time felt normal because of the hours of tense playing I was putting in. Tension and pain were simply present all the time and constituted my 'norm'. Suddenly, my playing started to actually deteriorate despite my diligent, daily practice.

In hindsight I could see that I'd tied myself into knots of tension with an unhelpful, overachieving attitude. I was unaware that

116 It is now called the Sydney Conservatorium of Music.

my focus was damagingly narrow and that I was practising an unhealthy way of being. My type A attitude was the root of my problems, affecting breathing and face muscles which are fundamental to playing a brass instrument. So I found myself at twenty-three years of age—supposedly a hot-shot player, who had studied at the Conservatorium, been a state finalist in the ABC[117] Young Musician of the Year competition,[118] played in professional orchestras—no longer able to play a note! I'd ground to a complete halt.

At this point, some months after applying, I learnt that I'd won a scholarship to do a postgraduate performance degree in Germany. But I arrived in Germany entirely unable to play. I spent months going from one specialist to another, trying different treatments. Finally I had myself referred to a neurologist in Harley Street in London. This man told me, 'If I were you, I'd look at a different career.' That was not an answer I was interested in.

As luck would have it, just before I travelled to London, a musician friend lent me *The Alexander Principle* by Dr Wilfred Barlow.[119] Dr Barlow was a rheumatologist and an Alexander Technique teacher, and while in London I went to see him. He said, 'Well, I don't know if we can cure your lips, but you could certainly improve the environment within which they have to function.' I started having lessons with one of Dr Barlow's co-teachers, Tessa Cawdron. I was quickly astounded at what Tessa showed me about what I had been doing to myself physically in the pursuit of perfection in playing music. Those years of dedication to becoming the best player I could be had resulted

117   Australian Broadcasting Corporation.
118   It was then known as the ABC Instrumental and Vocal Competition.
119   Wilfred Barlow, *The Alexander Principle: How to Use Your Body without Stress* (Arrow Books, 1975).

in an entrenched maldistribution of unhelpful tension. It involved elements I could recognise as they were pointed out. Maladaptive tensions had built up unconsciously over years; I had not recognised them and I regarded them as normal.

I had intermittent bursts of Alexander Technique lessons and, over the next year, learnt to leave out of my playing many of the tensions that had complicated it to the point of breakdown. Built-in tension had stopped me playing, so I had to learn to play without it. For the first two months, my practice consisted solely of bringing my instrument up to my lips without tightening my neck. It was clear that I was already good at tightening indiscriminately when lifting the trombone, so I needed to practise lifting it without undue tightening. There was no point in playing a single note that I didn't produce with the most freedom that I was capable of. This meant that initially I had to let go of the goal of playing at all, let alone well. Rather, I aspired to producing just one note freely. When I could play one free note, I allowed myself a second. It was a process of establishing a way of playing that did not include unnecessary tension. Recognising that I was the primary instrument which played the musical instrument, gradually, by making good use of my self, rather than playing, the primary goal, I rebuilt my playing with new foundations.

This indirect approach was the fastest and most reliable way of getting through my difficulties. It took about two years of paying close attention to my use to get back to playing at a professional level. I was able to complete the postgraduate performance course. After this, I trained to become an Alexander Technique teacher. During the couple of years of rebuilding my playing, my focus had shifted from playing to the mystery of how to change fundamental attitudes to achieving goals.

Like me, you also have a story that can be told in terms of the Alexander Technique. Make sure you can clearly articulate what you want your pupil or class to learn from your story. For example, in my story, I could focus on the type A, try-hard elements, which many overachievers can relate to. I could also highlight the process of undoing poor habits, unreliable sensory appreciation, the emphasis on the means, not the ends, or the fact that it was possible to come back at all from something for which the medical profession had no answers. You can tailor your emphases to your audience.

Sensation: Means, not ends

Don't encourage your pupils to seek sensation. Rather, help them to pay detached attention to it. Sensation is how we perceive the world—it is unavoidable. Detached attention does not mean ignoring sensation. It means being open to and registering, yet not judging, sensory information. Part of your job as a teacher is to help your pupil cultivate a useful attitude toward sensation—one of detachment as opposed to dwelling in it. This can help them identify and become more sensitive to key elements which influence everything else, for example, tightening the neck or holding the breath.

Both you and your pupil want to observe sensation with detachment. Your pupil may give you feedback that shows that they notice something, but at first, they don't know what element is important or worth giving attention to. Guide them to attend to the things that will help give them control over their use. Pick up points as they arise in the lessons and connect these points to each other. You can put the pupil's awareness in a context which you progressively build. Relate what they notice to their everyday life—this could be something simple like tying their shoelaces or reaching for a door handle.

If you ask your pupil what they notice, see if asking can occasion something about their use—connections or relationships between parts—becoming clearer to them. For example, you have just given them a table turn. Before your pupil gets off the table, you can lightly ask if they observe anything having changed. Asking at this point offers the pupil space for impressions to register at all. Articulating impressions helps the pupil conceptualise them rather than having them remain vague feelings. Often, what pupils notice is a consequence of the absence of unnecessary tension. Encourage them to connect a sensation of greater freedom with questions like, 'What have I let go of?', 'What am I now not doing that I usually do?' or 'How did I achieve that?' You may then have created an opportunity for saying to your pupil, 'Now we know that this freedom is possible for you' and, thus, perhaps inculcating some aspiration. Such understanding is what pupils take away to work with.

There is a risk in asking, 'What do you notice?' It is almost an invitation for the pupil to disappear into their physical sensations, losing the bigger picture that is available via detached self-observation. Vigilance is needed to head off any such tendency to rummage. Rather, encourage in the pupil neutral, dispassionate observation—an attitude of 'Oh, that's interesting and now let's renew the means that produced the result.'

Asking your pupil whether they have noticed something gives them an opportunity for self-reflection. This can throw up surprising and unexpected responses. I don't usually ask for feedback unless I am fairly sure, because I felt it with my hands, that something has changed. As a new teacher, with little perception of my pupils, I did not ask at all. Either way, discourage your pupil from getting attached to what they observe. Bring their attention to how they generated the experience, not the experience itself. Point out that grasping the how offers them the capacity to create it for themselves, putting the means in their control, not yours. Again, emphasise the means, not the end; the process, not the outcome.

What makes the Alexander Technique different?

If you are clear about what it is that you are teaching, that also clarifies the limits of your remit as an Alexander Technique teacher. Be sure of these boundaries. Step outside them very cautiously and with great circumspection. Do not be seduced by the wish to directly help someone or to solve a problem for them. Your job is to teach the Alexander Technique—'the control of human reaction' with reference to primary control relationships[120]—in whatever way you think is appropriate. Do relate what you have to offer to their problems and interests. But ultimately it remains your pupil's job to join up the dots in a practical way for themselves, connecting use (their responsibility) and functioning (the outcome). They have to engage their own will.

Keep in mind where the Alexander Technique differs from other means of self-help:

· It makes inhibition explicit;
· It is about the control of reaction;
· It asks for a particular quality of direction;
· It includes an explicit understanding of the integrated interconnectedness of use and function, i.e., primary control relationships;
· It remains free of attachment to a necessarily immediate outcome; and
· To teach it, you have to apply it.

---

120 Alexander, *Use of the Self*, 32–37.

As a teacher who continues to work on themselves, you develop. Your understanding matures. At every point in your career, assume that your experience of a primary control that is working well or poorly will continue to develop. You can transcend your experience and your level of understanding again and again. This will be reflected in how and what you teach.

Early lessons

The idea of working on yourself, i.e., having a choice in how you use your self and exercising that choice, is sometimes completely foreign to a new pupil. This is particularly the case for those who have bought into the model of medical intervention and of handing over responsibility for their problems to someone else. Often, these pupils come to you with a problem which they may have been seeking help with for a long time. With such a pupil, many lessons, particularly the early ones, may riff on how they can help themselves by using a skill they didn't know existed. You may have to emphasise to them that there are choices within their control, that they can improve their state, that this is their responsibility and that focussing on the problem is not the solution. As with any pupil, you are there to convey a way for them to work on themselves.

For the pupil to get anywhere with the Alexander Technique requires an attitude of practice. Ideally, you communicate implicitly or explicitly that your expectation is that your pupil is working on themselves, i.e., paying attention to how they use themselves in everyday life—exercising their own agency. Convey with your words that using the Alexander Technique is effectively a practice, even if you don't use this particular word. You might refer to it as body-oriented mindfulness or as a way of paying attention.

From every lesson after the first one, you can already be setting the scene with your initial greeting. It could be something like, 'What have you been working on?', 'What did you discover this week?' or 'How is your practice going?' versus the more open 'How are you?' This brief, initial conversation will give you clues as to how to proceed with the lesson.

It is important to get your pupil to attend to the positive, not to what hurts. Some pupils need to be coached to acknowledge what has improved, rather than clinging to what has not. After the first lesson, if you have demonstrated that it may be useful to pay attention to the relationship between their head and neck, and how to do so, many will start to notice tensions or interference.[121] Some pupils need to be told that this is not nothing. You can help your pupil realise that they are able to make a change (albeit probably a small one) and that this is not something they were able to do before they began taking lessons. Their ability to attend and steer a change for the better in the moment has broadened.

Having a little think in the morning about each of the day's pupils can be a useful part of preparing for each lesson. Create a picture of the overall arc of each lesson, yet be prepared to amend or drop your plan in the light of what they bring that day or what emerges during the actual lesson. In short, have an intent, yet don't be attached to it, nor to conveying everything at once.

---

121 Get them to notice that they tighten even more, or at all. Give them examples of activities where this might happen, for example, while doing up their shoelaces or reaching for something on a high shelf. If they notice that they exaggerate neck tension in any circumstance, then they have started to discern something that was previously opaque to them, and they can extend this discernment.

Teaching inhibition and direction

As a teacher, you need to ask yourself

- What in my pupil—beginner or experienced—constitutes the first element of present interference with their better use?

- How can I help this pupil understand their particular interference to greater freedom and expansion?

- What does my pupil need to pay attention to right now?

- What concept, image or story might help them?

- What is something that my pupil can consciously and voluntarily influence, even if just a little, which opens the door in the direction of general coordination and an experience of better use?

Examples of the last point might include an idea around not pulling their head back, allowing contact with the chair or that length is available. These considerations are generic. Your job is to make them relevant and specific to the particular pupil, leading them to the experience of better-organised primary control relationships. Where do you find a way into their pattern of use?

It is quite clear that if the pupil's back is to lengthen, the neck muscles which attach to the head can't simultaneously be shortening. Thus, for example, we usually start with some version of an intention for a free neck such that the head can orient forwards and outwards, relative to the top of the spine.[122] Or maybe, more realistically, we aim for the pupil to have less 'back and down'. Either way, this initial attention to the neck can rapidly ramify, because lengthening of the

---

122 See, for example, Patrick Macdonald, *The Alexander Technique As I See It* (Mouritz, 2015), 81.

back feeds straight into the 'up' of 'forward and up'—they are interlinked.[123] If expansion is to be coordinated, the traditional formulation of directions starts with the neck, for example, 'neck free', 'not to pull the head back' or 'let the head lead'. This is because any interference to freedom in the relationship of head and torso means the head is held in some version of 'down'. It is worth noting that for some people, freeing their neck may actually start much lower down in their back.[124] Thus, the pupil's experience of this first step may be in the realm of inhibition or in the realm of direction, depending on the pupil.

It is your judgement call as to what is going to engage and inspire your pupil. If your pupil has a new experience, you might name it. Help them understand that what is important is not so much the experience (which they may want to attach to) as how they got it.

Trust, elasticity and sticking to principle

As beginning teachers, often we don't trust our hands to convey what we want them to. This can persist for some time. Because we may not feel a clear response from the person under our hands, we worry that nothing is happening. But the more you don't interfere with yourself, the more trust you can have in your hands. Don't be attached to verbal feedback from your pupil, positive or otherwise. If you fulfil your end of the transaction, which is inhibition, your hands can have a profound influence and you may not know it at the time. There is always the risk of responding to a lack of trust in the process by trying to get the message across with little bits of 'doing'. If you feel under pressure, come back to basic principles. Let go of the need for an outcome. The more challenging you find

123 See 'FM's hands', page 43.
124 For example, see "Notebooks," in Stratil, *Irene Tasker*, 265–266.

your pupil, the more you need to stick to the principle of doing less. This is a perfect instance of the need to give primacy to working on yourself in order to be of use to anybody else.

If you want to convey 'up', length, breadth or integration, you need it in yourself first. This means coming back to your directions—your trigger or aide-mémoire—to refresh the sequence of ideas that results in elastic expansion in you. The quality of your use may convey an experience of integrated, elastic undoing if you have embodied this quality yourself. Otherwise, your work may be piecemeal, relatively unconnected bits, which Dilys Carrington referred to as 'just pulling people about—and that's not the Alexander Technique'.[125] However you express the quality of elastic expansion, it needs to include the direction of your head; the length, breadth and depth of your torso right into your pelvis; letting your torso balance up off your legs, whatever position you are in; simultaneously giving your weight to the ground while using the ground to release up off; and freedom for your breath. Practising this can become your way of being. And trust that this process will gradually help your hands 'hear' more.

Anxiety

A few years ago, a woman booked a first lesson. When she arrived, very flustered and somewhat after the appointed time, it was clear that she was quite an anxious person. Her anxiety was amplified by her being late. My first task was to help her calm down. I paid even more attention than usual to meeting her where she was, while remaining calm myself, and slowing my speech. When I eventually put my hands on her, this continued to be the theme—acceptance of her and how she was, while helping her to notice the chair under her,

125   John Nicholls reports Dilys Carrington often saying this in the 1980s.

bearing her up. I didn't try to 'teach' her anything. Gradually she calmed down and her breathing became deeper and freer. Then she was in a state to be able to attend to herself.

In my ears, during that lesson, I had Walter Carrington's advice to new teachers:

· 'You are not there to do anything to anyone!'

· 'Pay the closest attention to your pupil's breathing!'[126]

I would add this: be curious about what is interfering with your pupil's breathing.

Activities

Often, pupils compartmentalise their Alexander Technique practice from the other things they do, forgetting that the Technique is a tool to be applied to everything. Pupils often need help to make these connections.

Application work

Be interested when a pupil mentions that they do something regularly, for example, driving, gardening or holding a baby. This is an opportunity to help them connect what you are teaching them to what they do in the rest of their life.

Any activity can be used to demonstrate principles of the Alexander Technique. It is not, for example, about how to hold a flute, sit at a computer or perform a martial arts kata. The application is rather a vehicle for the pupil to learn about their use. Your understanding of apparently arcane Alexander procedures, like semi-flexion, sit to stand or the whispered ah, brings depth to working with pupils on activities. You can bring the underlying principles into any activity.

---

126 Carrington, *Thinking Aloud*, 47.

Then, you can further relate what you show your pupil to the context of daily life. For instance, if you have been helping someone who has a shoulder, arm or hand issue in relation to computer use, you might demonstrate that the same considerations in moving their arm apply equally every time they reach for a glass of wine, turn on a tap or pick up their toothbrush. You might need to improvise to simulate some activities; for example, you could use a small rucksack full of clothes as a substitute for holding a baby.

Fitness regimes

Keen exercisers tend to be dependable with their exercise routines. If you can help your pupil understand that they can apply the Alexander Technique while exercising, then their consistency with exercise can be even more positive, as they foreground their use while they exercise.

Get your pupil to show you what their daily fitness routine consists of. If it is something like a yoga practice, ask them to pick an asana and work on it with them. If it is a gym routine, you may need to improvise equipment. For instance, you could use a broom as a substitute for a weights bar. If you are working with a walker or a runner, ideally go outside and see what they do. If a walker uses walking poles, watch them using the poles.

As always, the emphasis is on how. You are there to support your pupil in appreciating how paying attention to their use — head–torso relationship, length, breath and ground contact — affects their performance. You are not there to critique their activity, but to help them with their use of themselves as they perform it. Stick to principle. Your criterion as an Alexander Technique teacher is primary control relationships.

Remedial exercise

Often, remedial exercises are approached with a degree of resentment at having to do them. Consequently, many people are not terribly diligent about how they do them, or doing them at all. They often stop doing them fairly quickly, so probably won't do themselves much damage even if they perform them poorly. But those who do keep up remedial exercises might as well perform them with the best use that they can muster.

When working with a pupil who is doing remedial exercise, you can encourage a shift of emphasis from the exercise to their use. Ask your pupil to show you what they do and tell you what instruction, if any, they have been given on how to perform the exercise and what its purpose is. The context of their use, utterly fundamental to good functioning, may be entirely missing from their understanding. Be circumspect about explicitly critiquing the idea of remedial exercise; rather, turn it into a vehicle for the pupil to practise using themselves well.

Ideally, having got your pupil to show you their exercise, gently guide them into doing it with less interference. From your Alexander Technique teaching point of view, you are helping your pupil move away from basic and fairly predictable interferences that are completely avoidable. Looking at the exercise in a lesson also provides a wonderful opportunity for you to reiterate the key idea that they are using their whole self, not just the bit they think they are exercising—no one part operates in a vacuum. This includes when the pupil is performing stretches, strengthening exercises and doing yoga. You are asking them to pay attention to what they are doing, as opposed to engaging in mindless repetition. At the very least, while performing an exercise, they have to support themselves against gravity and they have to breathe. Framing an exercise in these terms can help the pupil realise that they have the capacity to positively influence the quality of their exercise and its outcomes.

You don't have to say the words, but you can demonstrate, clarify and explain that tightening the neck, holding the breath or tightening the legs is not helpful. You could reiterate that in spending time on a supposedly remedial process, good use is foundational to the best outcome. You may also need to help your pupil realise that the sensory result may well feel different; for example, the sensation that they previously interpreted as a stretch may have been anything but. Or else they may be attached to feeling like they are working hard. Get them to notice how the outcome is more effective when they pay attention to their use.

Here is an example from my personal life: I was visiting my in-laws. My stepmother-in-law had fallen and broken her ankle. She showed me the mobilisation exercises that she had been given by her physiotherapist. I asked if she had been given any instructions on how to carry them out. Her answer was vague. Watching her, it was clear that as she flexed and extended her ankle, she was also unhelpfully tightening her lower back. I wanted to get her attention and I had a good relationship with her, so I provocatively said something that I would not say to a pupil: 'If you keep doing that you will end up with a sore lower back.' I then showed her how she could approach the ankle movements better. However, she continued performing the exercises without expanding her attention to include the relationships of one part to another. Eventually, she did indeed end up with a sore lower back. That finally got her attention!

Working with musicians

Here is a template for working with performers. It can be used with instrumentalists, singers or people in any activity.

Start by getting the musician to play or sing something simple that they are entirely comfortable with. It might just be a slow scale. This will give you an idea of how they use themselves with their instrument and provide them with a benchmark or starting point to compare with what may follow. Then get them to begin again, without the instrument.

Remind your pupil of the basics: the nature of the relationship between their head and torso, allowing the ground up through their whole body, that their whole torso is three-dimensional and that it breathes. The breath is one hundred percent accurate as an indicator of the state of the primary control relationships. Not interfering with the breath is just as important for a violinist, pianist, drummer or classical guitarist as it is for a singer, wind instrumentalist or brass player.

Even with an air guitar, air violin, reciting the words of a song or bringing the hands up onto the closed lid of the piano, you may need to get your pupil to stop and start again more than once as you help them stay in neutral. It may take picking up the air instrument several times before they realise that there is indeed something to pay attention to, connected to how they play or sing, which they can influence positively. You are helping them recognise unnecessary pre-playing muscular tensions. If these are present without the actual instrument, then the instrument is likely to be a much stronger stimulus to unnecessary tightening. Suggest that they prioritise attending to whatever element of their use that you think is most relevant at that moment. It should be something that they are capable of perceiving and steering for themselves. Don't be afraid to get them to rehearse, for instance, lots of air flute while attending to their length. Then challenge this by asking them to bring the actual instrument up as if to play. When they can do so with freedom, ask for a slow scale, a long note or something else they are completely comfortable with.

As you go through this process with your pupil, think about how you frame what you say. Not 'You're tightening your neck' or 'You are clenching your legs' but rather something along these lines:

- What would happen if you thought about what your head is doing as you bring the flute up?
- Do you think you could pay attention to your breath as you bring the violin up?
- What happens with your knees when you get ready to play a note on your trumpet?

Respect the expertise that musicians bring and the years of practice they have already put in. Don't make the pupil wrong and certainly don't make their instrumental teacher wrong! If necessary, ask them why they do something the way they do it. Attend to their primary control relationships:

- Do you think you could allow your neck to remain soft as you bring your hands to your guitar? (Simultaneously touch where you want them to think about.)
- Could you pay attention to your balance on your sitting bones as you pick up your drumsticks?
- What if we try it this way for a moment?
- What would happen if...?

There can be a great deal, going back many years, attached to the apparently straightforward act of playing an instrument.

This could include, for example, expectations from parents, teachers and self, memories of humiliating experiences, self-imposed pressure, pain, disappointment, unconscious beliefs, wanting to get it right, and trying to please the teacher. There are plenty of possible pitfalls around the artist's ego. Go gently. You may be opening a Pandora's box or even defusing a bomb, depending on the pupil's level of attachment to their beliefs. One pupil of mine, an accomplished musician, teared up just holding her violin as she inhibited her usual preparatory routine. Your pupil's trust in you, the teacher, is of vital importance. Be sensitive to their need for trust.

Flautist example

The following story demonstrates the importance of trust. With it, the professional flautist concerned was able to change a long-held belief about breathing. She came to me wanting help with shoulder and neck tension and pain. She was agreeable when I suggested keeping the first few lessons general, without her flute. (I wanted to be able to introduce the idea of good use without the pressure of playing.) After four or five lessons, I asked her to play me something she was comfortable with. I then asked her to put her flute down and mime the same thing. Predictably, she accurately replicated how she played. From what I could see, it seemed that to answer any questions about her neck and shoulders, we might usefully start with the breath.

I knew that this could have ended badly, given that almost anyone, and particularly a wind player, may have strong beliefs and attachments regarding their breathing. While bearing in mind that this pupil was an in-demand, highly competent professional musician, who had tens of thousands of hours of playing under her belt, I gently probed her thoughts about breathing. She revealed that a much-revered teacher had given her the image of a balloon collapsing as an analogy for breathing out. To me, this picture conveys active collapse — it worsens coordination and makes the next in-breath more difficult. This was, in fact, roughly what was happening.

With my hands on her, I encouraged her not to collapse. I asked her to breathe out so that she could start to understand and experience not only that she didn't need to collapse to exhale, but also that air could come back in more easily when she hadn't imposed collapse during the exhale. This demonstration was enough for her to realise that she didn't need to hang on to her old flute teacher's collapsing-balloon image. Not collapsing to breathe out also set the scene for her to be able to maintain a better relationship between her torso, shoulders and arms. This contributed to a positive effect on her neck and shoulders.

While I did not expect her lack of attachment to a long-practised misunderstanding, I was delighted at how quickly she was able to amend her use.

Singer example

A singing student, performing while standing, was tightening her legs as she sang. This was interfering with her ability to allow air in freely for the next phrase. She had already attended several group Alexander Technique classes and was familiar with paying attention to the relationship between her head and torso. With my hands on her, I asked her to release her heels down away from her bottom each time she wanted air and I reminded her of this each time. It was immediately apparent that releasing her legs made the next in-breath freer and easier. Simultaneously, she lost the harsh edge to her high notes and her sound generally became fuller, warmer and freer.

She repeated this experience under guidance several times in the class, until I was confident that she could replicate the process by herself. For her to develop this freedom in her breathing, she needed to practise the act of releasing overall, including down the backs of her legs, each time she wanted air. Initially this meant letting go of the need to adhere to the constraints of the musical pulse, and rather making a priority of practising the freedom to let air in. Before she could sing with the freedom she now knew to be possible, and according to the musical pulse, she had first to practise the freedom, and the facility to maintain it when under the pressure of the time constraint.

You have to take the process back to a point where the pupil can exercise the sort of choice you want them to bring into focus. Thus, for example, encourage the singer to prioritise developing facility with letting air in freely, detached from making a sound. For a singer, mastering the necessary intermediate steps requires letting go of what they may have previously learnt about breathing, or being overly focussed on singing the song. This is entirely possible in the practice studio, where student musicians spend most of their playing time.

General

It is always a judgement call about what to say and what not to say to a pupil, and in what sequence, whether they are a musician or not. This is also true of the sequence for leading questions and the giving of new information, for example, the idea that muscularly, the arms are rooted in the back, not in the shoulders. Or you may ask a question to get your pupil to think about and articulate something that they are experiencing. For instance, 'What effect is there on your breath when you don't lock your knees?' Answers to any questions you ask should, ideally, come out of the pupil's experience of a better state of coordination. This helps anchor the learning: if they can describe or explain it back to you, then you know that they have something they can work with. If not, this may lead to a further discussion or different approach to working with the pupil.

Some Alexander Technique teachers advise new pupils to stop playing their instrument for a while. My attitude, generally, is for my pupils to keep playing and use the challenge of remaining focussed on their use as an opportunity to learn. Their practice might, for a while, not involve making a sound at all. Your task is to make clear to your pupil how to practise using themselves well, definitely not how to practise their (demonstrated) problems. The flute player discussed previously was already competent at collapsing on her out-breath. She needed to develop even greater competence at *not* collapsing on her out-breath.

The pupil must understand that they are practising the use of their primary instrument: themselves. Playing a note should be secondary to and consequent upon good use. They need to practise the process of getting to the point of being *able* to play a note, such that a successful experience is more or less guaranteed. In lessons, you may need to take your pupil through this approach slowly, clearly and probably many times. Time on establishing good means is well spent since it makes everything else easier. This attitude needs to become part of your pupil's music practice.

Group teaching

After I had been teaching for about a year, I had the opportunity to work with groups of about eight people. Even more than in one-to-one lessons, I noticed how easy it was, with my inexperience and lack of practice, to get 'do-y' with my hands. I tended to 'pull people about', because I wanted something to happen, for them to feel something. If I was able to not take that tack, but rather just put my hands on and keep working on myself, that's when participants started to get an appreciation of inhibition or direction, usually far more than I was aware of in the moment.[127]

A key element is trust in the process. This requires that you apply what you know; don't get attached to an outcome; leave yourself alone; and avoid direct doing. Whether you are teaching an individual or a group, it still comes back to getting your own 'inner spring' going. If you are not elastically energised, you won't be able to encourage this quality in your pupil. This means dealing with nervousness: inhibiting anything that shrinks you, restricts your breathing or pulls you away from the floor; any need for a particular outcome; and whatever else distracts you from being present. To teach effectively, certainly to use your hands effectively, you need to provide an oppositionally active connection between the floor and your hands. This means allowing the floor to 'come up through you'; with free, responsive breathing, and opposition between your hands and everything else—back, head, floor and so on.

Building trust

Encouraging interaction and dialogue with and among your group helps build trust. You can ask carefully considered questions, usually open-ended ones, that give the participants plenty of space. As they answer, the participants should feel that you are listening and are interested in them.

---

127 They would tell me afterwards, or put it in the feedback form.

In a beginner group, you might ask

· Why are you here?

· What do you expect to get from this class?

· Assuming, for example, that people draw a connection between posture and pain: Why do you think posture has anything to do with pain? (This can lead towards the concept of use.)

Accept all answers. They give you an opportunity to steer the conversation and build in the group a shared understanding, direction of enquiry and language. If you need to 'correct' a misapprehension, or encourage a shift of emphasis, meet the comment with 'Yes, and...'. Never make the pupil wrong. Rather, gently guide them towards a more nuanced or sophisticated understanding.

Entertainment and games

When working with an individual, it is easy to have their attention. However, with a group you have to work a little harder to keep them all simultaneously interested. This means that at a certain level, you start as an entertainer—you have to engage them.

We learn best when we are having fun. Find instructive games or fun activities, ones that you like best.[128] Make sure that you can clearly articulate what you want your class to learn from the game or activity. Take time to explain the game. If people don't understand, ask what is not clear and carefully explain those parts again. Play the game, discuss the learning points and play it again.

---

128 For a great resource, see Rossella Buono and Anne Mallen, *For the Love of Games* (Self-published, 2017).

Planning a single group class or a series

Here are some basic questions you can ask yourself when preparing for a group class:

- Who is my audience?

- How can I most reliably teach them the Alexander Technique?

- What can I reasonably convey within the timeframe?

It is important to have an overall plan in mind for each class, with a clear beginning, middle and end. For a series of classes, consider a logical sequence of teaching points, to be covered over the series. Each class may have just one key learning point, which you highlight. You may touch on other points, but generally have just one key learning for each session. Think about how you might emphasise or summarise this key learning point at the end of the class. Don't overestimate how much the participants have understood or embodied at any time. Similarly, don't underestimate how much some random, throwaway line of yours may be remembered or valued.

Aspire to keep everyone involved all the time. If you use your hands as much as possible, as I do, on one person at a time, think about how you can simultaneously keep the rest of the group interested and entertained. Develop a repertoire of side demonstrations that everyone can participate in; these can relate to that session's particular point. You can encourage active observation. Anatomical or other explanations may be apposite, and stories can be useful.

Be precise with words like 'thinking' when what you mean is Alexandrian directing. Consider how else you can convey the idea of direction. For example, there are various games that can introduce the idea. I also always use affirmative feedback when I have my hands on and feel the pupil engaging their own direction. Emphasise and demonstrate that whatever experience they get with guidance in a class is within their reach to get for themselves. You are helping to prime them or wake something up which is already in their system.

Questions to the class are good. They promote interaction and make participants think about and articulate points to and for themselves; this supports learning. When you ask a question, get comfortable with waiting, giving time for people to answer—trust that they will. People's answers may tell you something about what they have or haven't understood, and what you may need to clarify. Likewise, questions from the class reveal what needs clarifying or explaining. Be prepared for unusual or strange questions. Sometimes I have found a useful answer may be, 'That lies outside of the scope of our topic.'

Be aware that dynamics will develop within any group. You may need to manage the people who dominate or draw out the quiet ones. A great way of helping the group form can be to ask participants to pair up or form groups of three, and then have them share with their partners about the previous activity. This fosters learning through having to think about what just happened and articulate it. It also provides a useful change of pace and activity, and can refocus the energy in the room. Later, sharing in the whole group can help people realise that they may not be alone in having the experiences they are having. This includes that of the difficulty in finding the words to describe new experiences.

When setting up the teaching space, be alive to the space and how it is or isn't working. Make it cosy and welcoming. You may need to move spare furniture out of the way or shift chairs into your desired formation. Consider the light: where is the window? You don't want to place yourself in shadow or where you become a silhouette.

Analyse and think through your performance after every class: what went well and what you can do better next time. This will facilitate planning for the next class and help hone your presentations over the long term. Of course, many of these points apply equally to one-to-one lessons.

Working with activities in a group

In any group, you may devote part of a class to getting participants in turn to bring forward an activity that they wish to work on individually.

- Ask questions;
- Respect the expertise of the participants;
- Get them to show you what they are doing first; and
- Go gently.

Take your time to understand why they may do the activity the way they do it. There may be a reason, good or bad, that needs uncovering. For example, many people pick up instructions about breathing from a choir conductor or a yoga or Pilates teacher. Such comments may have been misunderstood, taken out of context or taken to an extreme. They might have been ill-informed in the first place or even downright wrong.[129]

Online teaching

Online misses all the juice!

LK JOHN[130]

The information in this book on inhibition, direction, hands and how to build hands-on skills[131] remains relevant to online

---

129 See 'Activities', page 135; and 'Working with musicians', page 139.
130 LK John, personal comment to author, May 14, 2023.
131 See, for example, 'Inhibition', page 15; 'Direction: Intent and non-doing', page 22; and 'Hands, embodiment, repetition and attention', page 108.

teaching, because they are all ultimately about working on yourself; teaching means working on yourself. But the question remains: can we really teach the Alexander Technique online? Here are some thoughts and questions.

While I have taught online, I often find it unsatisfying. A judicious mix of online and in-person teaching may have its place, particularly for pupils or groups who have had in-person experience, for example, in places where there is no local teacher. A potential problem for those whose learning is mainly online, without direct, hands-on guidance, is that they cannot know what experiences they are missing: they do not notice what they have not encountered. This is particularly of concern for beginners.

In a hands-on lesson, as well as words, there is a sort of tactile conversation between the teacher and pupil which offers depth. Why else did Alexander use his hands?[132,133] Online, of course, it is limited to being a verbal conversation only. This means that online communication is purely conceptual, leaving potential pitfalls of faulty sensory appreciation for both teacher and pupil. The direct perceptual elements are missing, i.e., the teacher's hands receiving subtleties of real-time information about the pupil's use while communicating information to the pupil in person. Using hands, communication is direct, rather than being filtered through the medium of words, two separated nervous systems and computer screens. Notwithstanding having observation skills, answers to the following questions when using the hands can be clear and immediate: is the

---

132 See Barlow and Davies, *Examined Life*, 65. The period referred to was in Melbourne and Sydney, before Alexander left for the United Kingdom in 1904.

133 See Marjory Barlow, "Master Class with Marjory Barlow," *The Jerusalem Congress Papers: Back to Basics* (1999): 9.

pupil's use actually improving? Is their use being simplified and integrated through inhibition and direction? With hand contact, the teacher can listen and communicate directly.

It is clear that people can learn things online that are helpful. However, just because it is helpful and you have a teaching certificate, is it necessarily the Alexander Technique? For example, learning anatomy is fascinating, but it is not the Alexander Technique. Can a teacher lead their pupil towards freedom from deep habit via words alone?[134] The means of gaining new experiences rely fundamentally upon inhibition and direction. If they do not, then the method is probably not the Alexander Technique. The bottom line in teaching the Alexander Technique is to convey inhibition—preventing the wrong to create space for something else; and direction— waking up the primary control relationships.[135] Without the ability to touch, can we really convey to a person a different way of consciously being that asks them to work deeply with their primary control relationships?[136] Moreover, aside from inhibition and direction, the richness of what can be implicit in hand contact—integration, connections, calm, acceptance, support and encouragement—is likely absent while teaching online. Touch is powerful, and a well-trained, practised touch even more so.

---

134 See the comments about describing the colour red. Aldous Huxley, "A Psychophysical Education," in *More Talk of Alexander*, ed. Wilfred Barlow (Mouritz, 2005), 66. Also Alexander, *Constructive Conscious Control,* 77: FM quotes a friend, 'We cannot write a kinaesthesia any more than we can write the sense of sound.'

135 See 'Inhibition', page 15; and 'Direction: Intent and non-doing', page 22.

136 'I must emphasize...that knowledge concerned with sensory experience cannot be conveyed by the written or spoken word, so that it means to the recipient what it means to the person who is trying to convey it.' Alexander, *Use of the Self,* ix.

Pitfalls of hands-off teaching may include that

- It becomes a lot of 'doing' by both teacher and pupil;
- The pupil's interpretation of what the teacher is asking is not correct;
- The teacher is unable to detect and help with something that is going wrong;
- There is more possibility of the teacher being ineffectual;
- The teacher doesn't have to work on themselves— a fundamental of teaching the Alexander Technique— as consistently as when they teach face-to-face; and
- It can become a teacher's excuse to not develop their own hands-on skills.

Effectively teaching and learning the exacting skills of inhibition and direction in person is already a challenge. I would suggest that it is even easier to teach poorly online than it is in person. Because it is easy to get some sort of change in someone and for them to feel different, it is easy for both teacher and pupil to fool themselves—the change may be a disintegrative one and got through the wrong means.[137] An oft-cited plus of hands-off teaching is that indisputably, the pupil is the agent of their own change. However, is it stopping what's wrong? Online, can the teacher or pupil know that the change produced is one that simplifies and integrates use? Application of the organising principles of use, the primary control relationships, inhibition and direction are more difficult to verify remotely. Thus online work risks becoming something other than the Alexander Technique.

---

137 Because we are dealing with the use of the self, not posture, breathing per se or anything else we interface with, hands-off teaching tends to run a risk of some sort of stiffening or other misinterpretation of instructions, or otherwise missing the point.

If we purport to teach the Alexander Technique—the constructive conscious control of the individual—remotely, I suggest that the teacher's deep foundation in inhibition and direction is more relevant than ever. And even then, teaching online is still fraught with challenges. Yes, the pupil may own something more when taught without direct contact from a teacher's hands. But are they getting what they paid for?

Postscript

*In an era when all that is required to be acceptable members of
the chattering classes is to utter various shibboleths, James held
the line. He believed that you also needed to do your homework.*

GEORDIE WILLIAMSON[138]

How do we know we have adequately done our Alexander
homework, let alone done it well? Is it enough to stay in our
comfort zones, for example, our affiliations with training
lineages? How do we know we have transcended the intellectual
learning of FM's concepts and embodied them? Ultimately,
we probably don't. We need to be brave enough to leave our
'small bunkers of mutually reinforcing certainty'[139] and make
ourselves vulnerable to more learning. As teachers, can we
ever be aware of our own lacunae?

---

138   Geordie Williamson, "Home, James—Remembering a Cultural Giant," *The
Weekend Australian Review*, November 30, 2019.
139   Williamson, "Home, James."

Seek out opportunities for deepening your own practical skills and the understanding that ensues. Practically, you could find someone with whom you can regularly swap work. Speak respectfully and build trust. Keep challenging each other with questions. Work with your strengths and strengthen your weaknesses. As much as you do know, assume that you don't know everything. Theoretical frameworks, for example, knowing about anatomy or pain science, can be enlightening, but don't confuse conceptual frameworks with practical skill. Neither FM nor first-generation teachers had current theoretical knowledge about physiology or interpersonal communications. What they had was the ability to use their hands to gather information about their pupil and reflect it back.

It is comfortable to rest on our laurels, and not progress beyond a certain point in skill and understanding. Similarly, it is all too easy to mistake insights for mastery, learnings for understanding, technical skills for real ability and words for their meanings. Embodied knowledge and practised skill in self-application provide ever-deeper foundations for teaching. It is hard to overstate the importance of continuing to deepen our knowledge of, and skills with, the basics. Competence in the basics is our bottom line. Peggy Williams'[140] advice is apposite: learn to do the simple things well.

140   Peggy Williams (1916–2003) was trained by FM Alexander.

Acknowledgements

I am deeply grateful and offer heartfelt appreciation to:

My many teachers, including Tessa Cawdron, Inge Henderson, Jeanne (Day) and Aksel Haahr, John Nicholls, Carolyn Nicholls, Anne Battye, Adam Nott, Jean Clark and many others;

Those, all encouraging and helpful, who battled through early drafts and those who read later versions: Alex Kaufman, Ann Shoebridge, Malcolm Williamson, Ruth Rootberg, Merran Poplar and Polly Keightly;

Colleagues and students who have endured many discussions, and obliged me to greater clarity;

My patient and supportive editor, Dayita Nereyeth and my inspired designer, Tess McCabe;

And last, but not least, my greatest supporter, partner in life and work, Léonie John, who keeps me on track.

About the author

Michael Stenning is a former orchestral musician turned Alexander Technique teacher, who teaches privately and trains teachers. He has taught all over the world and offers professional development to both new and experienced Alexander teachers with a disciplined yet informal approach. Michael is a former Chair of the Australian Society of Teachers of the Alexander Technique. When not teaching he enjoys walking in the mountains, backcountry skiing and photographing nature. Michael lives in Canberra, Australia.

www.freedominaction.com.au

www.ingramcontent.com/pod-product-compliance
Lightning Source LLC
Chambersburg PA
CBHW051258020426
42333CB00026B/3258